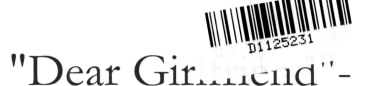

"Dear Girlfriend"-

A Handheld Walk Through Breast Cancer

SUZAN RIVERS

ISBN-13: 978-1482512571
ISBN-10: 1482512572

TO CONTACT SUZAN RIVERS:

www.facebook.com/suzan.rivers.1

www.amazon.com/author/suzanrivers

www.smashwords.com/profile/view/suzanrivers

For Walker

Special thanks to:

Lynda and Skip Woodall for their constant encouragement,
direction and editing.

Aaron Glaze for his powerful cover art.

Vicki Molnar for being such an enthusiastic and energetic Media Coach.

CONTENTS

I AM SO SORRY. YOU POOR THING. YOU POOR POOR THING.

Dear Girlfriend,

You don't know me, but I know you. You have been diagnosed with breast cancer. I am writing this to help you, and to help myself, survive breast cancer. This is my own true story. I hope it will help to give you peace of mind. So here I sit at my kitchen table, with a cozy fire in the fireplace, writing to you, my new girlfriend. Here is my gift to you, my story of survival....

I was diagnosed with breast cancer in December, 2008, right before Christmas. What a Christmas present! Now it is November, 2012. Having breast cancer has been one of the worst things, and oddly enough, one of the best things, that has ever happened to me. I keep thinking that if I can help just one other woman get through breast cancer with a few less tears, and maybe a few more laughs, then all that I have been through will not have been in vain.

Fighting cancer is not only about healing your body because you are not just a body. You are a duel being. You have a body, but your body is just the vehicle in which your soul dwells while you are here on earth. Fighting cancer is about healing your body and restoring your physical beauty, finding peace of mind, and learning to really believe that your soul is eternal, so that you can understand more fully what it means to be a human being. When you have accomplished all four of those goals, then and only then will you feel truly cured.

Have you ever seen the movie *Harvey*, starring Jimmy Stewart? If you have not then I strongly suggest that you go out and buy a copy. This is one funny movie and God knows you need to surround yourself with as much humor right now as possible! In this famous comedy, Jimmy Stewart, who plays Elwood P. Dowd, has an unusual friend. This friend is an invisible white rabbit, named Harvey, well over six feet tall. Elwood talks to Harvey all the time, so of course most people are convinced that Elwood has lost his mind. Elwood's sister, Vita, gets so embarrassed by her brother talking to Harvey, that she makes arrangements for Elwood to be committed to a lovely little mental asylum called Chumley's Rest.

So to make a long story short, Dr. Chumley, the psychiatrist at Chumley's Rest, tracks down Elwood to have him locked away because of this rabbit named Harvey. Then the unthinkable happens. Dr. Chumley starts seeing Harvey. He realizes that Harvey is not an hallucination and Elwood P. Dowd is not crazy.

Dr. Chumley likes Harvey so much that he wants Harvey to leave Elwood to come stay with him. Poor Dr. Chumley. He has spent his life trying to bring peace and tranquility to his patients who come to stay at the lovely Chumley's Rest. But who can bring peace of mind and tranquility to poor old Dr. Chumley? Elwood P. Dowd is so sweet and understanding; he even listens to Dr. Chumley's troubles as Dr. Chumley lays out on the psychiatrist's couch in his own office.

Dr. Chumley tells Elwood that all he really wants is to go to Akron, Ohio. He wants to lay his head in the lap of a beautiful, mysterious woman who will give him beer to drink, listen to his troubles and console him.

Now what I want to say to you is that it is okay for you to feel like you want to be consoled. You are a woman, so I know that you have consoled many people in your life. You have been there to console your husband, your children, your aging parents, your friends. Now you have been diagnosed with a life threatening disease. Now it is your time to be consoled. You have to be open and willing to accept the love and consolation of your family and friends in order to survive cancer. You have to be open to the love and healing power of God in order to survive cancer. I am fifty-six years old. I grew up in the days when women were bombarded with the notion that we had to be strong. Inner strength is great, but now is not the time to shut yourself off from people. Now is not the time to prove that you can fight this battle on your own. Now is the time to face the fact that even if you live on this earth until you are one hundred years old, that is really not much time left. This life on earth is very temporary, but you must remember that if you have faith in God, life is eternal.

Right now you are afraid, but I'm hoping and praying that I will be able, with God's help, to show you how to conquer your fear so that you can put all your strength and energy into getting well. Yes, you have been diagnosed with a life threatening disease, and yes, it is okay for you to let someone hold you and pat you and tell you how sorry they are that you are going through this mess.

When I found out I had cancer, I called a very close friend of mine to tell her my devastating news. I suppose she thought she was saying the right thing when in a very optimistic, chipper voice she said, "Oh, you'll do just fine! Millions of women have been through this... You can get a cute wig and it won't be bad... You'll do just fine!" I wanted to slap her head right off her shoulders! I didn't want to hear about the millions of other women who have had breast cancer. I couldn't take on saving millions of other women. At that moment I was in survival mode. My life was being threatened, just as threatened as it would have been had I stepped on a rattlesnake or been kidnapped at gun point and thrown into the trunk of a car!

If you have been diagnosed with cancer, then you know that your fear is just as palpable as it would be if you were being chased around the room by an axe murderer. When you are experiencing this kind of fear, when your body goes into the panic mode, when you are walking through the valley of the shadow of death, you don't need to hear, "I'm sure you'll be fine!" because there is really no way that your friend can be sure that you will be fine. You want to scream, "Stop telling me that I'll be okay because you don't know that I will be okay!!! You don't know what's going to happen to me!!!"

There. Now I've said what you want to say to your friends or husband or lover so that you don't have to say it. If you do say it, then they will just be hurt and confused and back away from you when you need them to be there for you more than ever before. Think of me as your new best girlfriend. Girlfriends get us through this life. I want to be your girlfriend. Imagine we are sitting in our favorite little coffee shop at a table for two. You have just told me the most devastating news of your life, "I have cancer." I take your hands across the table and I say, " I'm so sorry that you're having to go through this. I love you so much and I don't know much about this thing, but I'll try my best to help you get through it. If you want to scream or cry or throw things, I'll make sure you don't break anything too expensive...." Then you will smile a little through your tears and I'll give you a paper napkin to blow your nose and say just one more time, "I'm so sorry. I'm so so sorry...."

KEEP TELLING YOUR FUNNY STORIES.

Dear Girlfriend,

My big dream is that my breast cancer story will help you survive breast cancer. I guess if we are going to be friends I should tell you a little about myself. My name is Suzan Rivers. Right now, because I have recently been in the process of breast reconstruction, I am not working outside my home. When I am working, I am a librarian in an elementary school. I am happily married to Walker Rivers. He is a private consulting forester. He helps people take care of their land and forests. We have three daughters in college.

I'm going to tell you a story about how we came to live in Macon, Georgia, in a huge old mansion nestled behind two of the biggest magnolia trees in the state. You are probably wondering what that has to do with breast cancer. Everything. You will see. Everything.... So take your mind away from your diagnosis and enjoy this story. I am an old house person. Since we married thirty six years ago, Walker and I have always lived in an old house. We moved into the historic district of Macon, Georgia, in 1984 and bought a house built in 1911. We restored the house one room at a time and brought home three baby girls while we lived there. We loved our little home, but Walker decided that he wanted to have his office in the house, so we started looking for a bigger old house to buy.

That's when we discovered that 923 High Street was about to be sold to a local church and they were going to tear it down for a parking lot. I was aghast! This six thousand square foot Classical Revival house had twelve huge Ionic columns, a balcony and a solid marble front porch. The old part of the house, the kitchen, that I am sitting in right now as I write to you, was built in 1840, and the "new" part of the house was built in1879. The first family to live in this house raised seven children here. This old home has so much history that the thought of it being torn down for a parking lot just made me sick.

I had heard through the grapevine that the lady who owned the house had already sold it to the church for demolition, but I just had to go talk to her anyway. I just had to save that house! That was in 1996. At that time I had three beautiful little girls. Laurel was seven and her identical twin sisters, Olivia and Blythe were six years old. I had made arrangements with Mrs. Jordan, the owner of the house, for us to come see it. Mrs. Jordan was soon to be ninety and had lived in the house for fifty years.

As it just so happened I had taken my little girls, the night before, to see The Nutcracker Ballet. They were the most impressed with the scene where the Rat King is stabbed to death by the Nutcracker. Oh silly me... I thought they would be impressed by all the sweet little girls dancing around in their beautiful costumes. Nope. The next day, the day we were supposed to go meet Mrs. Jordan to see my dream house, my dainty daughters spent the day reenacting over and over the same scene from the ballet, where the Rat King is stabbed to death by the Nutcracker. I just shook my head as I watched them run around the house taking turns on who would get to do the stabbing and who would get to be the dying rat. Oh well... girls will be girls!

So when Walker got home from work, I got my three little darlings all dressed up like Shirley Temple. They had on their cutest little frocks, adorable little patent leather Mary Janes, and each of them wore a huge red bow in her hair. They looked just precious, lovely...well, you get the picture. Then we loaded up the car and headed to 923 High Street. When we got out of the car, I straightened their hair bows and smoothed their dresses and said, "Okay girls, Mommy wants to buy this house. If we don't buy this house they are going to tear it down. Just look at these huge magnolia trees!" Three little heads looked straight up. " Now, you don't want those trees and this house to be torn down do you?" Three little heads shook "no". "Okay now, I want you to be on your best behavior. I want Mrs. Jordan to see what good little girls you are." Three little heads nodded "yes". As we walked up the marble steps, three little heads stared up at the twenty-five foot tall columns. All the columns were covered with thick vines. There was hardly any paint left on the house. Walker leaned over and whispered in my ear, "Have you lost your mind?"

We rang the bell and Mrs. Jordan opened the door. She was a teeny tiny little woman but she was very healthy and had a certain feisty air about her that I liked right off . "Come in! Come in! Oh, what pretty little girls. Twins?"

"Yes ma'am," I answered.

"Oh, I have twin daughters too. They grew up right here in this house!" Three little heads nodded. She walked us all through the house. I must admit it was a diamond in the rough. It had been divided into five apartments. Every square inch of the house needed major work. Of course in my mind I was already picking out paint colors, wallpaper, and where to place the furniture. "Would you like to see the staircase?" Mrs. Jordan asked the girls. Three little heads nodded "yes". She took us into a back room where there was no staircase and said, "Isn't that a wonderful staircase?" I thought, "Oh great. She's gone 'round the bend...." Three little faces just looked confused. Then Mrs. Jordan went over to the window seat, threw off the pillows and lifted up the seat. There it was. A hidden staircase! Three little faces just smiled.

We walked back into the living room and Mrs. Jordan said,"Well, what do you think?" At that my oldest daughter Laurel said, "Would you like to see us be dead rats?" I thought, "Oh, nooooooo!"

Mrs. Jordan said, " Yes. I would love to see you be dead rats." Then all three of my babies lay on the floor and started to kick their legs up in the air with petticoats flying. Then they all, as if on cue, held their "paws" up in the air, turned their faces towards Mrs. Jordan, hung their tongues out of their mouths, rolled their eyes back and said, "Bleeeeek!!!!" Then they died.

Walker and I couldn't help but laugh because we knew exactly what they were doing, but poor Mrs. Jordan didn't have a clue. I held my breathe for her reaction. She burst into a big smile and started clapping. "What wonderful dead rats! I love it!" I breathed a sigh of relief. Walker actually shot me a look to let me know to go for my dream house. I said, "Mrs. Jordan, we really want this house. If you sell it to us, I promise we won't tear it down. We'll fix it up and raise the girls right here."

Mrs. Jordan said, "I'll be happy to sell it to you. It needs these little girls...I mean these little rats, to grow up in it." So we left, and when we got outside the girls asked, "Did we do good, mommy?"

"Yes! Yes! You did so good. You were perfect. You were just perfect!" Walker seemed to have warmed up to the notion of restoring the house, and we were all excited and happy as we drove away.

Now, I guess you are wondering what that cute little story has to do with cancer. Absolutely everything. Listen to me. Cancer can't steal your stories, not if you refuse to let it. Cancer can't steal your funny, happy memories that have shaped your life and made you who you are. Cancer can't steal the love of your friends and family. Concentrate on that and you will make it!

> **Girlfriend advice: Tell your funny stories. Keep your sense of humor. Make your family and friends laugh. Look cancer in the face and say, "You can't take whatever it is that makes me myself. You can't take my spirit. You can't take my soul. I will live forever and there is nothing you can do to change that!"**

WELL, YOU HAVE CANCER.

Dear Girlfriend,

I want to tell you my story, but what worries me is, how can I tell you what I went through having breast cancer without scaring you? Having cancer is scary. Having your breasts removed can be traumatic. It was traumatic for me. So should I sugar coat this story? Should I try to downplay the fear and trauma that I have experienced or just tell you the real truth? I want to tell you the truth. When you have cancer you really do need to be guarded about what you read and what you let people tell you. The heart of my story is that cancer can cause fear and suffering, but for millions of survivors, it is only temporary. What comes after is a new you.

This new you will have learned to live each day to the fullest. This new you will love and forgive everyone in your life as if it were the last day of your life on earth. This new you will have no time for petty conflicts. This new you will choose carefully who you want to spend time with. You will find it easy to push all "poison" people from your life. You will never let yourself get talked into being on some volunteer board or president of the neighborhood association unless you really, truly feel like doing it. You will realize that this stage of life on earth is short. You will resolve to spend the rest of your life, even if you live to be one hundred, doing what you really want to do, with the people you really want to be with.

Of course there will be days when you still feel afraid, or down in the dumps. I still feel anxious or depressed at times, but, overall, I like the new me. Most important of all, this new you will hopefully come to the conclusion that there is a life after this incredibly short life on earth and that stage of life is eternal. Yes, cancer can end this stage of life on earth, but fear not, cancer can not take eternity from you.

Where do I start? When I was just sixteen years old I found a lump in my right breast. It was surgically removed and found to be a benign cyst. Ten years later at age twenty-six, I found another lump in that same breast. I had it surgically removed and it also was found to be a benign cyst. The surgeon who removed those two benign cysts told me that women who have cysts in their breasts rarely get breast cancer. I don't know if that is actually true or false. What he said gave me a lot of relief, but probably made me careless about doing breast self examinations. You should check your breasts at least once a month, right after your period, so that you can detect any changes.

Fast forward to the year 2008. I was working in an elementary school as a librarian. When I got off work in the afternoons, I would generally run errands. I started to notice that I was so tired I just couldn't make myself do those errands. I would go to the grocery store and just sit in my car with my head down on the steering wheel thinking, "I can't do this. I can't get the groceries. I can't lug them up the steps into the house. I can't cook supper. I can't...I just don't have the energy." So, I would just go home and crawl into bed and go to sleep. My husband, Walker, would cook supper for my daughters who were seniors in high school.

As the months dragged by I just felt more and more tired. Now, I have a wonderful gynecologist who I have been seeing for many years, but no matter what she tried, I still felt wrung out all the time. I decided to go to see a specialist, a reproductive endocrinologist, to see if anything could be done about my constant fatigue. He put me on a bio-identical estrogen. That was in August of 2008. Then one morning at breakfast in December 2008, just five months later, my husband Walker said, " Last night when we were in bed... I...uh...I felt something in your left breast." I didn't feel particularly alarmed because I figured that it was just one more of those benign cysts. " Well, I'll get it checked out," I said nonchalantly over the top of my coffee cup.

Then I started thinking that maybe I should have been doing those breast self exams, but I hadn't. The reason I hadn't been doing them was because twice in the distant past I had found a lump, and even though it had been so many years ago, whenever I did a breast exam on myself, it made me feel very queasy. I guess I was just so afraid that I would find something bad, that I rarely could bring myself to do a breast self examination. Let me tell you something, I was so stupid to not check my breasts every single month. If my husband had not accidentally felt that lump right when he did, if I had not gone to my gynecologist right when I did, then I would probably be dead today. Ladies, please, I cannot stress to you enough, how important it is to check your breasts every single month for the rest of your lives.

If you have never done a breast self examination, this is the proper way and, yes... it can be a little scary the first time because you are afraid you will find something. Go in your own bedroom, lock the door, and lie on your bed without your bra. Raise your left arm over your head and let it rest on the mattress above your head. Take a deep breath and let it out. Relax. Now take your three middle fingers and rotate them gently all over your breast. Chances are you will feel nothing but soft tissue. I have found that if you put a little lotion on your fingers then they will glide over your skin making the whole process easier. After you examine your left breast, do the same on your right side. If you do feel something hard, something that feels different than the other side, then you should call your gynecologist and ask her to see you as fast as she can. Don't let some receptionist tell you that the next available appointment is in a month, insist that you get an appointment now.

Now, let me tell you this, according to my gynecologist, eighty percent of all breast lumps are benign. So don't freak out if you find a lump, but don't be an idiot either. Go to your doctor and get it checked out. The right time to do a breast exam is right after you finish your period. Do it at the same time every month so that you can note any changes. If you are post menopausal then decide what day of the month you will do the exam and mark your calendar for the entire year, like the first day of the month or the first Friday etc.

Back to my story. After Walker told me he had felt "something," I went in my room and did a breast examination just as I described. I felt the lump. It was about the size of a green pea. I felt a little queasy but went right to the phone to call my gynecologist, Teri. I didn't have to beg for an appointment. Teri's nurse, Corrine, had the receptionist make an appointment for the very next day for me. I felt very loved and cared for because she was so understanding. She knew that I was scared and she wanted to get the exam over with quickly so I could stop feeling afraid. I should have sent her a thank you note, but I didn't. My bad. Let me tell you that over the course of your breast cancer treatment you will meet many angels. Nurses and doctors and technicians appreciate your letting them know that they are appreciated. Send them little thank you notes or small inexpensive gifts and you will be amazed at how much that will mean to them. By the time you finish this journey, they will all feel like family to you.

The next day I went to see Dr. Teri Luhrs, my very competent and caring gynecologist. She was optimistic and reminded me that she had done a breast exam on me just five months earlier, before the reproductive endocrinologist had put me on bio-.identical estrogen. Five months earlier Teri had felt nothing in my breasts. So I put on the lovely paper gown and climbed up on her examination table. She started to perform the exam as we chatted away and then she felt it. She didn't miss a beat. "Oh, I feel what you felt. This wasn't here in August. Listen, eighty per cent of these lumps are benign, but I'd like for a surgeon to look at you." I felt my first little tiny bit of fear. "Just put your clothes on and meet me in my office," she said. While I was getting dressed I was thinking about my relationship with Teri. She was my doctor but she had also been my neighbor and close friend for over twenty years. She had lost her first husband to cancer. She knew that time was of the essence if one is going to survive cancer.

So I put on my clothes and walked down the hall to her office. I thought that in all the years she had been my doctor, she had never asked me to come to her office. I felt a twinge of queasiness. She sat down on one side of the desk and I sat on the other. "Do you have a surgeon in Macon that you feel comfortable with?" she asked. "Dr. A removed my gall bladder. I liked him," I answered. So she called Dr. A and made an appointment for me for the next day. "Now, don't worry. It's just better to be safe than sorry. It's probably nothing," she said as I walked out to the waiting room.

The waiting room, as always, was full of pregnant women. I had never been pregnant. I had used fertility drugs for six years but they didn't work.

I wondered if all those hormones could have given me cancer. I had never birthed a child. I had never nursed a baby. I wondered if not using my female parts had caused me to have breast cancer. I had adopted my three girls when they were babies, but I could not have loved them anymore if they had come out of my own body. Thoughts. Thoughts. Thoughts. Had I done something wrong that caused this lump? Could I actually have cancer this time? No way. I was sure that it was just one more cyst.

When I got home Walker asked, "Well, what did she say?"

"Oh, she said it was probably nothing, but she made me an appointment with Dr. A for tomorrow."

"I want to go with you."

"Okay."

The next day I was right back in a doctor's office. Filling out forms. Filling out forms. Filling out forms. You better make doggone sure that you have someone listed that your doctor can release information about you to in case you do have surgery, or else your doctor will not talk to your husband or friends or family while you are still out cold from anesthesia. The laws about patient privacy are there to protect you, but you need to give your doctors the name of someone to talk to, about you, or you could be waiting around for many hours before your doctor can personally come to talk to you in the hospital.

The doctor that I had come to see was a general surgeon who had taken my gall bladder out a few years before. He was not a surgical oncologist, but he was very competent and very nice. The first thing he did was a physical exam of my breast and then an ultrasound. If you have never had an ultrasound, let me tell you, there is nothing to fear. An ultrasound is painless. Your doctor will put some lotion on your breast and then rub a wand that will remind you of a microphone, around on your breast. The ultrasound sends high frequency sound waves through your breast. The waves bounce off the lump in your breast and the image of the lump can be seen by your doctor on a display screen. This image will also be recorded on X-ray film. Your doctor can look at these images to help determine if your lump is just a fluid- filled cyst or a cancerous tumor. After my doctor performed my ultrasound he said there was something there that was not just a fluid- filled cyst.

He said, "I think we need to do a needle biopsy. I'll just numb this area of your breast using a local anesthetic that I'll put in with a needle. Then I'll insert another needle close to the lump and extract a few cells to be examined. This won't hurt a bit." He then gave me a shot of painkiller in my breast.

Girlfriend advice: There is no reason for any medical procedure you have performed on your cancer journey to hurt.

The doctor, even though he was very sweet and very kind, did not use enough local anesthetic to numb my breast. I should have spoken up as he put the second needle in to do the biopsy and said, "Wait!!! That really hurt, will you deaden it a little more?" If I had opened my mouth and told Dr. A that he was hurting me, he would have numbed my breast more, but I didn't say anything. My husband, Walker, was sitting at the end of the table I was on. He told me later on that he could tell I was in pain because I was holding on to the edge of the table so tightly and my toes were scrunched up so tightly.

When Dr. A had finished poking around inside my breast with a needle, I sat up and playfully said, "Liar! Liar! Pants on fire!" He just gave me a confused look and said, "What?"

"You said that wouldn't hurt, but it hurt really bad," I replied.

"Why didn't you tell me to stop? I would have numbed it more. I didn't mean to hurt you." Then he said as sweetly as anyone could have ever said anything, "I think you probably do have cancer, but we will get you through this. You are going to be just fine. We have to get these test results back and do another kind of biopsy, a core needle biopsy and a diagnostic mammogram. That's a mammogram that we use after a lump has already been found, but don't you worry, you are going to be okay."

Then he told his nurse to make the phone calls to arrange for me to have a diagnostic mammogram. His nurse said, " I can't call today." Dr. A gave her a stern look and said, "Do it today." The nurse looked irritated and left the room. I had the feeling that she was going to be hard to deal with, but all I could think about were Dr. A's words, "you probably do have cancer." As Walker and I walked through the front office the nurse said, " I'll call the breast center tomorrow." I thought, "Why wait until tomorrow? Why not call now? The mammogram place is still open, why not call now?" But just like with the painkiller, I didn't speak up. I didn't complain. My mother had raised a polite daughter....

Walker and I live a short distance from this doctor's office. When we walked outside, I felt so light-headed that I had to hold on to his arm while we walked home. I couldn't believe the words I had just heard. I kept holding on to the word "probably." I told Walker, "He said it was probably cancer. He didn't say that it was for sure cancer. Right?" Walker just said, "That's what he said."

"But you, you don't think it is, do you?"

"Let's just wait and see what these other tests say before we get all worried. Okay?"

"Okay." I had said okay, but I was already starting to get scared. For me, fear has been the hardest part of my journey through cancer. This was in December, 2008. When we got home, my beautiful house was all decorated for Christmas, my favorite time of year. I went into the front parlor where my twelve foot Christmas tree was loaded down with hundreds of ornaments that my three daughters and I had put on. We had just that year swapped out the little tiny lights for the great big colored lights that made the tree look like something out of the nineteen fifties. On the highly carved rosewood Victorian piano, I had placed the antique chalk ware nativity characters that Walker had bought for me for my birthday in a junk store in Savannah. They were each about twenty inches tall and extremely heavy. I had been so excited when we bought them. They had come out of an old church in England. I had had so much fun with my girls as we set out Mary, Joseph, Baby Jesus, the angels, wise men and the animals. We had surrounded them with greenery and red poinsettias. We had woven little white lights all around them. Laurel, Olivia and Blythe had made fun of the statues because they were so big. They had started calling them "the giants" and made up goofy names for the wise men.

We had had so much fun and now the fun was over. All the Christmas spirit had left me. I was cold. I curled up in a blanket on the couch in front of my Christmas tree lights as my daughter Laurel came in and started playing Christmas carols for me on the piano. I smiled and told her they sounded beautiful, but I didn't hear a thing. Nothing. Nothing except those words ringing in my head, "You probably do have cancer...."

For the next three days I called Dr. A's office to see if my appointment for the diagnostic mammogram had been made. It had not. We are talking cancer here, not a Brazilian butt lift! My mother had raised me to be polite, not stupid. I picked up the phone and called the breast center myself. I was told that an appointment for a diagnostic mammogram had to be made through the doctor's office. I explained that the nurse in the doctor's office was supposed to make the appointment, but she had not done it. The receptionist said she would call the nurse at Dr. A's office and make the appointment for me. A few minutes later the nurse at Dr. A's office called me and said, "Why did you call the breast center? I told you I'd do it."

"Well, you didn't do it. Look, I haven't slept a wink since I left your office three days ago. Waiting to find out if I have cancer is torture. I'm sorry, but I think I need to find another doctor." I hung up. I decided that even though I liked Dr. A and thought he was an excellent doctor, I wanted to get a different doctor. If dealing with his staff was going to be that difficult, I couldn't handle it. Looking back on it, I should have told Dr. A what happened with his nurse. At the time I just couldn't handle the stress of any conflict, and I didn't want to get his nurse into any trouble with Dr. A. My job was to find a good doctor who had a good staff that made me feel that they were competent and just as important, caring. How was I supposed to find this doctor that was just right for me? I didn't know where to turn.

I called a friend of mine who is a physician. He suggested that I go to a particular surgeon. My friend set up an appointment for me which was just five days after my going to see Dr. A.

Doctor "B" had a good reputation as a surgeon, except that several people had warned me that his bedside manner was not particularly warm. Walker again went with me to see Dr. B. As I sat on the examination table in that thin paper gown waiting for the doctor to come in, I was cold and scared. I didn't know what to expect, but I was expecting better than what I got. Dr. B breezed in without a trace of a smile to put me at ease. No comforting words, he was all business. I don't think there is a doctor alive that really, truly realizes how uncomfortable it is to have some man that is a total stranger come in and immediately start handling your naked breasts. It is embarrassing and humiliating, not to mention scary if you know there is a suspicious lump in your breast. This doctor just didn't seem to care. He finished his exam and said, " I'm going to send you down the hall for a diagnostic mammogram and a core biopsy."

Then he just turned around and walked out. I just sat there on the table wondering what new and ingenious ways of torture awaited me. At that point, a very friendly and talkative girl came to escort me to have the mammogram When we got to the mammogram room she gave me a nice warm terry cloth robe to put on. That robe helped me feel so much less vulnerable. Little things like that can make all the difference. While she did the mammogram she started jabbering away about all the problems she was having with her boyfriend, "You just wouldn't believe what my boyfriend did last weekend!" she said as she slipped the robe off as little as she had to while she took the pictures of my breast. Of course her story about her boyfriend kept my mind off what she was doing and that made me relax. She even made me laugh!

In case you have never had a mammogram, a mammogram is a kind of X-ray. Instead of taking pictures of bones, it takes pictures of tissue, breast tissue. A screening mammogram is the type of mammogram used yearly to look for lumps. A diagnostic mammogram is just used when a lump has already been detected. It takes pictures that zero in on the suspicious area. I stood in front of the machine while the talkative technician placed my breast on a tray. Then another tray came down on top of my breast to flatten it out while the X-ray was taken. It was not painful, but acutely uncomfortable. Somehow this young technician prattling on about her sorry boyfriend made the whole experience a lot easier. Some women might have thought she was being unprofessional, but I really appreciated her style.

Then she walked me down the hall to another room for the core biopsy. At that point she was joined by a female radiologist. I told the radiologist, "I don't really know what a core biopsy is, but I had a needle biopsy the other day at Dr. A's office. He is a wonderful doctor, but I didn't tell him that he was hurting me so badly that I wanted to jump out the window." The radiologist said, " You should have spoken up. Listen, this is not the dark ages. There is no reason for any of your procedures to hurt. I'm going to numb up your breast with so much painkiller you won't feel anything. Work with me here, if I hurt you, let me know, and I'll numb you up some more. Okay?"

All I could manage to say was, "Okay." She numbed my breast using a needle but it didn't hurt. Then she explained to me what she was going to do. "Okay! A core biopsy is a needle biopsy that uses a needle that is just a tad bigger than the needle Doctor A used on you. Instead of extracting cells, I'm going to use this needle to extract tiny bits of tissue. My helper here is going to guide me on where to insert the needle using the ultrasound and you and I both can watch the screen to see what's going on. Okay?"

"Okay."

She inserted the needle and I watched as she sucked up tiny bits of tissue into the needle. My breast was so numbed that I didn't feel anything at all. She kept asking, "Are you alright? I'm not hurting you, am I?"

"No. I'm fine."

When she finished, she showed me a little bottle of liquid that had the tissue samples in it. "See, this is what I extracted. These samples are called cores. I'm going to send them to the lab and they will determine if you have any abnormal tissue. So now we just say our prayers and see what happens."

"Okay." I felt like all I could manage to say was "Okay. Okay. Okay." I got dressed while the technician continued her boyfriend story. I felt like I was in the twilight zone as she led me back into the examination room where Walker was still waiting on me. I got dressed. We went home. In a couple of days we got a call from Dr. B's office saying we needed to come in for a consultation. That's when the fear factor started to rise. I figured that if I did not have cancer, the receptionist would have just told me the good news on the phone. I figured that I must have cancer.

When we arrived at the doctor's office, we were taken back to the examination room. I had a glimmer of hope because I figured that if he had bad news, he would break it to me in a nice warm office, the way they do it in the movies. No such luck. Dr. B breezed in. He didn't pull up a chair beside me. He didn't hold my hand or put a reassuring hand on my shoulder. Walker and I were sitting in two chairs side by side. Dr. B just crossed his arms as he leaned back against the examination table, "Well, you have cancer." That's all he said. He just stood there looking at us. I said, "Well, Merry Christmas."

Then Dr. B said, "How much do you value your breast tissue?" I didn't know what to say. I felt like he just didn't get it. I had never thought about my breasts as merely "tissue," like a wort or a mole.... I felt like he had taken that part of me that made me feel feminine and sexy and pretty and trivialized all those feelings by calling my breasts "tissue." I wanted to say, "How much do you value your penis tissue?" but there again, I was polite. I said, "I value my breasts very much, but of course I want to do whatever I need to do to stay alive." Dr. B said, "I can't give you one more day of life by taking off your breast. You will have just as good an outcome by just having a lumpectomy."

By the way he worded that sentence, I wasn't really sure how much of a chance I had to live. He said he would have his receptionist set up an appointment for me to have an MRI. He left. I asked his nurse if I could have a prescription for anxiety because I could tell my heart was racing and my head was starting to hurt really badly. She went to get the prescription while Walker and I just sat there in silence and shock. She came back with the prescription. We left.

I can't even begin to describe how I felt. As we walked out onto the sidewalk, cars were whizzing by. Birds were singing. People were walking down the sidewalk talking and laughing. A dog was barking in the distance. I just couldn't figure out how everything was just still going on as if nothing had changed in the universe, when I had just been told that I had cancer. I wanted to push a button and make the whole world just stop while I at least caught my breath and tried to adjust to this blow that had just been dealt me...

Girlfriend advice: We know that some breast cancer is estrogen driven. The question that I asked was, is there some sort of test to determine if you are one of those women who should not take estrogen because it may give you cancer? The answer to that question is no. However, if you have any of these factors that might possibly increase your risk of getting breast cancer then you may want to consider not using estrogen.

Some of these factors are:

if you have a family or personal history of breast or ovarian cancer

if you started your menstrual periods before the age of twelve

if you had a pregnancy, before the age of thirty, that you were unable to carry until birth

if you are obese

if you have a history of blood clots or stroke

if you have never given birth or nursed a child or had your first child after the age of thirty

if you have been through hormonal fertility treatment

if you consume more than one drink of alcohol a day

if you have a sedentary lifestyle

The long and the short of it is that the decision to use estrogen should not be taken lightly. Have an in depth discussion with your gynecologist before you take estrogen. If by not taking hormone replacement therapy you might possibly be lowering your chances of breast cancer, then maybe you should decide to just deal with the unpleasant aspects of menopause, such as hot flashes. Discuss all of this with your doctor before jumping onto the estrogen bandwagon, which could possibly increase your risk of breast cancer. I think it is also worthy to note that according to the National Cancer Institute : "a number of studies suggest that current use of oral contraceptives {birth control pills} appears to slightly increase risk of breast cancer among younger women. However, the risk level goes back down to normal ten years or more after discontinuing oral contraceptive use." So if you are planning to use birth control, it might be a good idea to talk to your doctor about your using other kinds of birth control instead of oral contraceptives.

CANCER GIVES YOU NO TIME OUT.

Dear Girlfriend,

Having cancer doesn't allow you to have time out. I remember running around outside playing chase or hide and go seek when I was a little girl. When one of us kids needed a minute to catch our breath we would holler, "Time out!" Time out was sacred. None of the other children would argue if somebody cried time out. We would all bend over and put our hands on our knees and breathe hard. Somebody would turn on the faucet on the side of the house and hold up the hose pipe for us all to get a drink. Sometimes the game would change to playing in the cold water from the hose. But cancer doesn't let you have one second of time out. There are people all around you that need you to still be you. Your husband, your children, your elderly parents, even your dog still wants to be scratched!

Your life, your story, keeps going on in full swing. Nothing slows down. I repeat nothing slows down at all! On that December day when Dr. B said, "Well, you have cancer," my world just kept on going. My world completely changed, but it didn't slow down for me to adjust to the change. So many things that I thought were so important, like working on the restoration of my house, were just not important anymore. Feelings that I had never had before flooded me. The feeling of fear and anxiety flooded me. I hated for the sun to go down... I could not scream, "Time out!" because I had to host a Christmas party four days after my diagnosis. I still had to do all of my Christmas shopping. It was up to me to make Christmas this incredibly memorable time for my husband, my children and my elderly mother who always comes to spend the holiday with us. How was I going to act like everything was fine and wonderful so that everybody at my house would have a holly jolly Christmas?

Then I remembered that old saying, "fake it 'til you make it" and I decided that was all I could do. I simply made a decision that I would not bring everybody down with my cancer. If I let cancer ruin Christmas for my family, then "Cancer" would win. I would not let Cancer win. I would pull off that Christmas party, do the shopping and the wrapping and the singing carols at the piano in the parlor. I would go to church to celebrate the birth of Baby Jesus with my husband and children. I would watch *It's a Wonderful Life* and *Christmas in Connecticut* snuggled up with my family in the TV room on Christmas Eve. I would wake up my three girls on Christmas morning and make them sit with me on the top step of the staircase. Then I would say to their daddy, "Go down and see if Santa Claus came!" And he would go down to the tree, plug in the lights and holler up the stairs, "Go back to bed! So sorry girls, he didn't come this year!" And then my girls, who were all grown up now, would laugh and run with me down the stairs because we knew he was lying. We would do it the same way we had always done it because I was not going to let my enemy "Cancer" win.

I decided that I would cook Christmas dinner and use all the same recipes that I used every year. I would make that same old apple salad that the girls would refuse to eat, and they would tease me about how awful it is. I would wonder once more, how many years it would take for them to catch on, that the only reason I make it, is because I love to hear them tease me about how awful it is. I would make sure everything was done for Christmas just like it had always been done. I would not let my family down. All of this I decided on the way home from Dr. B's office, but how in the world was I going to pull it off?

When Walker and I got home, my house was buzzing with the laughter and back- and- forth banter of three carpenters, Karl, Kyle and Patrick. At that point in time we had lived in our house for twelve years. We had kept our promise to Mrs. Jordan, the lady who had sold us the house. We had not torn it down. We had raised the "dead rats" in the house and had been restoring it one room at a time. When I was diagnosed with cancer, my twin daughters were seniors in high school, and my oldest dead rat was already gone off to college.

Over the past twelve years, Walker and I had turned the dilapidated apartment house into one of the most beautiful old single- family homes in Macon. The house had actually been featured on the national television show, "If Walls Could Talk." We had ripped out apartment kitchens from the World War II era. We had rebuilt the central Victorian staircase that had been torn out years ago to cut up the house into apartments. We had put back the kitchen as close as possible to what an 1800's kitchen would have looked like. We put two huge free standing antique dish cabinets in and kept the built in cabinets to a minimum. We left the 1840's fireplace where the original cook would have worked over a wood fire. We refinished the primitive pine mantle and slave made bricks on the wall behind it and put in gas logs to cozy up the place. We bought an exact replica of an old wood stove that is really gas and electric.

In 1842 the house where the famous poet and flutist Sidney Lanier was born, was built on our lot. In 1879 that house was jacked up onto huge logs and dragged by oxen to the lot next door, leaving the detached Lanier kitchen behind. In 1879 the main body of our house was built, and around 1903 the old detached Lanier kitchen was finally attached to the main body of the house. So in my kitchen the water was boiled to help with the birthing of Sidney Lanier.

Oh! That reminds me of something. You know how in the movies when a woman goes into labor somebody always hollers, "Quick! Go boil some water!" Walker and I were at my brother John's house when his wife, Carla, went into labor with their first baby. We hurried them out the door in great excitement. Then we went back into the kitchen to make some coffee. There on the stove was a huge pot of boiling water. We just cracked up! "John knew what to do!" Walker said. We have teased John for thirty-five years about that pot of water, but he always insists that he was just going to make grits. Ha! Likely story!

See, like I told you at the beginning, cancer can't take your stories...can't take your memories...can't take away what makes you you.

Getting back to the house.... When Walker and I walked in the front door from Doctor B's office, our carpenters were putting on the finishing touches to what had turned out to be an eight month long project. They had started in May of 2008 to finish the house. I had lived in that house for twelve years with five totally decrepit bathrooms. The "master" bathroom was a big box that had been built to stick off the side of the house on the second floor. Shortly after we moved in, I sat in the bathtub, praying that it wouldn't fall right through the floor. It didn't fall through the floor, but when I pulled out the rubber plug, I could hear the sound of water hitting leaves on the ground below. Yikes! All the other bathrooms had their own peculiar personalities. My daughter Laurel's bathtub would get air in the pipes so badly that the whole tub would shake while the pipes made eery sounds. She was afraid to use it because she thought it was haunted! We all still make fun of her for having a "possessed" bathtub.

For the first twelve years that we lived in the house we had only ancient floor furnaces and gas logs for heat in the bedrooms. I remember every morning in the cold weather, my three little girls would run down the stairs and get as close to the floor furnace as possible to stay warm, while they took off their nightgowns and put on their clothes for school. Most of the house had window unit air conditioners. Walker and I slept in an upstairs bedroom that had no air conditioner. It really wasn't bad. I'd take a cool bath in the haunted bathtub, open up the French doors in our bedroom that led out on to the balcony, point an old oscillating fan right at the bed, lie down, and if I didn't move a muscle, it was right tolerable. I actually liked it because I could hear the sound of trains in the distance. I loved that sound. Whenever I heard a train whistle blow, I would say a prayer for the engineer. I would wonder who he was and what he was thinking about as he drove on through the night. I wondered if he could feel my prayers....I'd fall asleep....

In May of 2008 we decided to bite the bullet and finish the house. You can't imagine how important finishing this house was to me. We had the outside painted, had a top of the line heat and air system installed and we had Karl, Kyle and Patrick gut those five bathrooms and rebuild them to perfection. By December of 2008, Karl, Kyle and Patrick had become part of the family. They had a ring side seat to everything that went on at the Rivers house. I made their coffee every morning. Kyle and Patrick were two good looking young men in their twenties. Karl was like a grandfather to Patrick. Their finishing up my house was just about one of the most exciting things that had ever happened to me. My dilapidated old house that was going to be torn down in 1996, was going to be ready to host

Macon's downtown historic district's Christmas party on December 13, 2008.

Walker and I had married in 1976 when we were both just nineteen years old. I had waited thirty-two years for this day, the day I would have a completely finished, completely furnished home, the home that I was sure I would grow to be a hundred years old in.... Then everything about the house that was important to me changed. Just a few short days before I was to host a party for the entire neighborhood, to show off the finished product of twelve years of many individuals' hard work, all of my joy, excitement and anticipation of a long and full life with my family in our beloved home was stomped flat when Dr. B leaned up against that examination table and said, "Well, you have cancer."

I know I can't possibly put this in the right words, but I'm going to try. You see, I had thought restoring our home was important. So very important. In the few seconds it took Dr. B to say, "Well, you have cancer," I looked back over my life at all the things I had spent time on and realized for the first time ever, that time is the only thing we have here on earth, in this stage of our eternal life. You see, up until the time that I was told that I had cancer, I never really thought about how short this stage of life on earth is. I thought I had all the time in the world to restore a house or a hundred other projects that take time. I thought all those very time consuming projects were so important.

Then I was forced to realize that my life on earth was like the hour glass that the wicked witch in the *Wizard of Oz* turned upside down. Dorothy saw the sand pouring through the hour glass and realized that her time was limited.... Now, what I am trying to tell you is that you probably will survive breast cancer, millions of women do survive breast cancer, but even though you survive cancer, your time on earth is limited. Please don't let that scare you because you can live forever, but life on earth does not last forever. Life on earth is short even if you live to be one hundred.

When I found out that I had cancer, I realized very fully, for the first time, that my life here on earth is so brief. I looked back at all the time I had wasted on unimportant pursuits. I looked back at all the conflicts with people that I could have avoided. I looked back at all the sins I have committed and I felt so much regret. I knew that I could never go back and relive my life on earth again, but I also realized that I didn't want to waste one minute of the time I had left here on earth. Time was absolutely all I had, and for the first time I fully realized that time here on earth is so so so limited and so so so precious.

All of this ran through my head in the time it took to get from the doctor's office to my house. So many of the things I had thought were so important, like restoring my house, were just not important anymore. Like the old saying goes, "You can't take it with you." There was only one thing that was important to me, staying alive, so that I could spend my time with the people that I loved the most, my family and my friends. I couldn't care less about working on my house or anything else, all I wanted to do was live so I could show my love to the people I loved. Everything had changed. I was in survival mode. I prepared myself for the fight of my life.

I remembered years ago when Walker and I went to Florence, Italy. We went to see Michelangelo's statue, *The David*. If you have never seen it, I promise it is worth a trip to Italy to see it. In this stone statue the young man David is depicted as he would have looked staring up into the eyes of Goliath . He has his sling shot over his shoulder and there is no mistake about what he is thinking. David is looking up at the giant Goliath thinking, " I am going to kill you. I will win this fight. You are going to die!!!"

I feel that all of us who are faced with cancer must feel like David. He had all the strikes against him. He was so much smaller than Goliath. He was not a soldier, but he had faith that God would protect him against all odds. And God did. Now my challenge, when I was diagnosed with cancer, was to hold on to my faith and believe that God would protect me. But on the day I found out I had cancer, even though I had promised myself to pull off Christmas the same as ever, and I had made all those plans that my faith in God would help me to hold on to, by the time I got home from the doctor's office I found that I couldn't hold on to anything at all....

When I walked in the front door that day and heard my carpenters, Kyle and Patrick laughing and talking, I didn't say a word. I don't know what my face looked like, but I remember Patrick's young, exuberant, smiling face when he said, "You okay? Is something wrong?" I just stopped dead still, and for the first time, I uttered those ghastly words, "I have cancer." And for the first time I saw what saying those words to a friend or loved one has the power to do. His face just changed so dramatically before my eyes that he didn't even look like himself. His eyes opened wide and his lips parted slightly. He looked as if he was aging right before my very eyes and in a sense he was.... He looked like he wanted to say something, but just didn't know what to say. So he said nothing. My ghost floated past him into my bedroom where I shut the door and lay on the bed. I longed to hear the sound of the train, but the French doors were closed. The new heating system blocked out the sound of anything outside my bedroom. I curled up on the bed in a small ball. I pulled the covers completely over my head....

BE AS OPEN AS YOU CAN ABOUT YOUR CANCER.

Dear Girlfriend,

Two days later was Friday, time for the "Bible Gang." The Bible Gang is a group of women who have been meeting at my house every Friday from September through May for fifteen years. The group started when the secretary of St. Joseph's Church asked me to host a group of women for five sessions of study during Lent in 1997. I only knew one of the ladies before the group started. At the end of the five weeks we all had grown to be friends. We decided to keep meeting on Fridays for a while longer. That was fifteen years ago. Two of our original members are in heaven, no doubt about that. Two had to drop out because of their jobs, and one moved to Virginia. There are six of us left: Caroline, Helen, Mary, Lisa and Lily. It took us fourteen years to read the Old Testament! So, you can tell we spend a lot of our time together talking and eating, but most of all laughing. Walker says he can always tell if the gang is in the house because we laugh so loudly. We yack about everything from recipes to sex. We have grown to love each other and we have become a support group for each other. I think that is just exactly what Jesus would want us to be doing.

These ladies, through their support of me, and each other, are actually doing what Jesus said to do, not just reading about it. These women met my daughters when they were just tiny children and now my daughters are grown. These women have given me advice on everything that a woman can possibly go through for fifteen years. Now they are looking over the boys that are coming around to date my daughters. Mary tells my daughter

Laurel, "Put all those boys in the cupboard! Go have fun! Enjoy yourself! I didn't get married until I was twenty- eight. You're too young to get married. Just put all of those boys in the cupboard and when the cupboard is full, you pick the best one, the one you want to marry. Your cupboard isn't full yet! Keep dating different ones!"

The "Bible Gang" is always there for one another. Our ages range from fifty-two to ninety-two, but we still refer to ourselves as "girls." The reason for that is that people always feel young on the inside. I believe that is because we are dual beings. The body ages, but the spirit, or soul, is eternal and so it doesn't age. On the inside, all of us are twenty and hot. Very very hot!

The day after I was diagnosed with cancer, I had to decide whether to be very open about my having cancer, or very hush hush. I had known women who withdrew from everyone when they were told that they had breast cancer. I had known other women who were very open about their cancer diagnosis. I felt that the women who did not withdraw from the world, but were very open and honest with people about what they were going through, fared much better than those who locked themselves away and tried to handle breast cancer privately. I think that some women are very hush hush about their breast cancer because they are embarrassed, especially if their breasts have been removed and their reconstruction has not yet been done.

I decided to be very open about my cancer diagnosis. So on that Friday I waited to tell the gang my bad news until they were just about to leave my house. I didn't want to throw cold water on what had been a particularly fun visit. When they were getting ready to leave, I said , "Hey y'all, I need to tell you something." They all sat back down and I had to say those awful words out loud again, "I have breast cancer." It was just like when I told my carpenter, Patrick. Seeing their fear scared me, but then they were all over me with hugs and well wishes and promises to pray for me.

If I had kept my diagnosis to myself, I would have missed out on all their expressions of love, and believe me, it has been expressions of love that have gotten me through this ordeal.

Girlfriend advice: Be as open as you can about your breast cancer diagnosis, as open as you possibly can. If you let people know what you

are going through, you will be blown away at how kind and caring people can be.

After the gang left, I called my sister, Cea, and told her to spread the word in our family about my cancer to everybody except Mama and Daddy. I didn't want them to worry about me. I told Cea to ask everybody she told to pray for me.

THAT'S SUPPOSED TO MAKE ME FEEL BETTER?

Dear Girlfriend,

The next day was the day of the Christmas party for the neighbors. When it was time for me to get dressed I stood staring into my closet. I took out a black cocktail dress that was very low cut. I held the dress up while I looked in the mirror and thought, "Well old friends, this is probably your last party." I put on the dress with the plunging neck line showing off my size 34D chest....

The party went just fine. The only memorable event was when one of my Catholic neighbors, who had heard about my cancer diagnosis, came up to me and handed me a holy card. " You just read this everyday and you'll feel better," she said. In case you don't know, a holy card is just a little card with a beautiful picture of Jesus or the Virgin Mary or maybe a saint or an angel on one side and a prayer or a poem on the other side. When the party was over I went up to my bedroom with the holy card still in my pocket. I took it out and read it and just started laughing. I picked up the phone and called my sister, Cea, in Virginia. I was laughing so hard I could hardly breathe. "You won't believe what just happened to me! This friend of mine just gave me a holy card with this poem on it that she said would make me feel better. Listen to this, just listen to this."

"I'm listening." I can't remember the exact words, but it went something like this, "The Lord is with you everyday... He listens when you kneel to pray... And when you are on your death bed dying... All alone, alone and crying... He will take away your pain... Like sunshine after pouring rain...As you close your eyes to die...He will take you by and by..."

"That's supposed to make you feel better?"

"Yes! Can you believe that? Isn't that a hoot?"

"That's the funniest thing I've ever heard!" Cea and I just howled with laughter.

"How in the world could she have thought that would make me feel better?"

"I don't know. That's the most morbid thing I've ever heard in my life!" she said. I was laughing so hard that the tears were just pouring down my face.

"Well, I better go ...I hope Jesus doesn't take me away tonight!"

"Yeah me too. That was so funny! Don't waste your time alone and crying..."

"I won't. Talk to you later...Bye!" I got in bed next to Walker and let him read the holy card. He just laughed. Then he said, "You've got to admit though, reading this card really did cheer you up. This is the first time I've heard you laugh since this whole mess started..." What he said was true. The holy card really had cheered me up. I actually felt better. I curled up next to him and said my prayers, " Dear Lord, thank you for giving me this card. I feel like you had something to do with it being given to me. I've been praying so hard to feel better and now I do feel better. You really do work in mysterious ways. And Lord, I think you must have a really great sense of humor! Nightie night...."

Sad to say that feeling better did not last. Over the next week my emotions were getting pretty much out of control. Let me tell you something, if you get diagnosed with cancer, don't feel embarrassed or ashamed to ask your doctor for medication for anxiety and depression. My most difficult emotion to deal with was fear. Fear of surgery and fear of death crept into my being and would not let go of me. If I could manage to fall asleep, I would wake myself up with the sound of my own scream. Needless to say, this was more than a little disconcerting to poor Walker.

He would be awakened by the sound of this terrible, primal sound coming from me. He would grab me while I gasped, "I can't breathe! I can't breathe!" Of course I could breathe because I was talking, but I felt like someone had their hands around my throat, choking the air out of me. When Walker managed to convince me that I could breathe, then the crying would start. I would just cry from sheer terror. I can best describe it as the feeling one must feel right before being executed. I cried uncontrollably as I curled up in Walker's strong arms and said, "I feel like I'm standing in line waiting to be hanged!"

Poor Walker didn't know what to do. He needed his sleep as much as I did because since he is a forester, he had to get up at five o'clock every morning to do hard physical labor out in the woods. I researched these horrible attacks on the internet. It gave me great comfort to learn that I was not losing my mind. This level of anxiety is quite common in women who are battling breast cancer. Every woman is different and every woman has her own set of feelings to get under control. I am no doctor, but I felt like my fear was coming out in my sleep because I was trying so hard to not be a "Gloomy Gus" during the day.

During the day I was on the "fake it til' you make it" program, because I didn't want my daughters and other family members and friends to be brought down, right there at Christmas, by my expressing the torment I was feeling on the inside. Since I wouldn't express all the terrible feelings I was having during the day, I would wake myself up screaming during the night. Some women have the personality type that if they are miserable, they want everybody around them to hear about their misery. I guess if they are suffering, they want to make sure everybody around them is suffering too. I wanted my friends and family to have a warm and wonderful Christmas, so I tried to hide my feelings during the day, but those feelings of terror were coming out in my sleep.

People have always described me as friendly, upbeat, and funny. So when I was diagnosed, I decided to just keep on being friendly and funny, even though on the inside I was scared past the point of description. Fear was my Goliath that I had to find a way to kill. I went to my primary care doctor for antidepressants and medication for anxiety. Depression and anxiety are not the same thing. Depression is overwhelming sadness. Anxiety is overwhelming fear. I experienced both, but I experienced more fear than sadness. Sometimes I would just cry and cry. I was crying because I was afraid, not sad.

Some women have uncontrollable anger when they receive their breast cancer diagnosis. Some women find themselves on an emotional roller coaster of crying from fear one minute and screaming from rage the next.

I have had a lot of anger in my life, but cancer did not make me angry. It just made me feel afraid to a degree that I didn't know I could feel. My fear was so intense that I really can't even describe it. The meds did help me to feel better, and, girlfriend, if you are miserable with fear or sadness, please get some medication to help you get through this difficult time. There is nothing to be ashamed of if you take antidepressants or medication for anxiety. If you don't do it for yourself, then do it for your loved ones, especially your husband. Walker was the only one I was being truly honest with about my mental misery and pain. At one point he actually said, "You need to tell somebody else how you really feel. You're only dumping all this mess on me and I can't take it anymore!!!" Hence this book. I can be honest with you, dear girlfriend. Together we can slay the Goliath of fear and depression.

THE MRI- MAGNETIC RESONANCE IMAGING

Dear Girlfriend,

So I got on meds to help control my emotions, and on December 19, 2008, I went to have my first MRI. If you have never had an MRI then you have nothing to fear with this procedure. MRI stands for magnetic resonance imaging. This test takes a more detailed look at your breast abnormality, especially if you have dense breast tissue. Sometimes even a diagnostic mammogram will not detect breast cancer if you have dense breast tissue. An MRI also helps your doctors to determine if you have cancer in other parts of your body. Now, waiting for the results of this test can be very stressful, but the procedure itself is not bad.

Before I describe the MRI procedure, I want to give you a heads up about insurance. On the morning that I went to have my MRI, I filled out the necessary forms at the imaging center and as always gave the lady behind the desk my insurance card. I asked her if the imaging center participated in our insurance network. In the good old days before cancer, when all I ever experienced were routine medical visits to my doctors, this line of questioning was enough. Either they worked with my insurance or they didn't. This time the lady behind the desk assured me that my insurance was good there and I needed to do nothing else. WRONG!

Unknown to me, certain large ticket procedures required pre-certification. That means that the doctor who ordered the MRI or the MRI center should have contacted my insurance company in advance and gotten prior approval for the procedure. Neither my doctor nor the center did this, and the receptionist at the imaging center didn't catch the fact that the procedure had not been pre-approved, even when we asked if our insurance business with her was in order.

The upshot of all this was that I was stuck with an MRI bill of $3600, since the insurance company refused to pay for the unapproved procedure. I later negotiated with the provider to reduce the fees in light of their blunder, but it still proved to be a costly lesson for me.

Girlfriend advice: Check, recheck, and check again with your health care providers and your insurance company well in advance of treatments.

Now, getting back to the MRI... an MRI does not use X-rays. An MRI uses a powerful magnetic field and radio frequency pulses to make pictures of your internal body. This can include bones, soft tissues, and organs. The technician who performs your MRI will look at the images on his computer monitor and then copy them to a CD that will be sent to a radiologist for evaluation. You can ask for copies of the CD to be sent to any of your doctors and keep a copy for yourself if you want a copy. An MRI does a more accurate assessment of what is going on in your body than an ultrasound or a diagnostic mammogram. Sometimes cancer is not detected by a screening mammogram or even a diagnostic mammogram if you have dense breast tissue. If you have been told that you have dense breast tissue I think an MRI would be money well spent, especially if a mammogram does not detect a lump that you can feel.

An MRI can help your doctors "stage" your breast cancer. Staging is a system that your doctors use to determine just how advanced your breast cancer is. An MRI can help your doctors determine whether or not your breast cancer has moved on to other parts of your body. That information will help you and your doctors plan your course of treatments.

After I finished filling out forms in the front office of the imaging center, I was taken back to put on the lovely hospital gown. The kind woman who escorted me back just happened to be a friend of mine. Any time you are helped by someone you actually know, it makes everything so much better. Seeing a familiar smiling face makes all the difference in the world. After I put on my gown and removed all my jewelry, my friend handed me over to a technician. The technician was very sweet and explained that for the MRI images to be seen clearly on the computer screen, she would need to give me contrast material intravenously. She started an IV on me and helped me get up into the MRI machine.

In the past, MRI machines made some people claustrophobic because they were placed inside a large tube that was closed at both ends. Now the open ended MRI is commonly used. It looks just like its name implies, it is open on both ends. Once in the machine I lay down on my stomach with my breasts hanging down in an opening in the machine. I had to stretch my arms out in front of me with my face resting on a padded frame that was quite comfortable. The technician kept saying how important it was for me to remain absolutely still. She didn't have to worry about me being a wiggle worm because I did not want to repeat this little procedure. Next she gave me earplugs because the MRI machine makes a terrible racket. It sounds like BANG! CLANG! BUZZZZZ! over and over again. If I hadn't been warned ahead of time, I probably would have scooted right out the end of that contraption half naked because it sounds like it's about to blow up or something!

Here's a good piece of news. The MRI does not compress your breasts like a mammogram does. Yippee!!! I had very large breasts so I hated mammograms. Taking something as big as a cantaloupe and mashing it as flat as a pancake is not comfortable. I'm telling you girls, the mammogram machine had to be invented by a man. An MRI is so much easier. There is no physical pain or discomfort unless you have an aversion to getting the contrast material intravenously. If that is the case, talk to your doctor about taking the contrast material orally. And now that the machine is open on each end you should not feel claustrophobic. If the fire alarm goes off you can just scoot right out of that thing. No problem!

So let's review. I was lying flat in the machine with my arms stretched out in front of me. My face was lying on a comfortable padded frame. My breasts were hanging down in an open area of the machine. The IV was in my hand, but it was not hurting. The earplugs were in my ears. The technician pulled out one of my earplugs and said, "Push this button!" Then she put something in my hand as she replaced my earplug. I thought to myself, "If I push that button will I blast off? I feel like I'm in some kind of spaceship." I started to hear BANG! CLANG! BUZZZZZ!!! I got up my nerve to push the button. All of a sudden all I could hear was Bing Crosby singing "Mele Kalikimaka", the song about how to say ""Merry

Christmas" in Hawaiian. I thought, "Holy moly! Can this get any weirder?"

The technician left the room, but she could see me through a window while she worked the MRI machine and talked to me while the pictures were being taken. I could hear her say, "Okay, Suzan , I'm going to release some contrast and you are going to have the sensation of coolness." I just stayed still and didn't say anything. The whole procedure took about an hour. When it was over the technician said, "You did good! Hope you like Bing Crosby. Now the computer will process the pictures showing thin slices of your whole torso. You can get dressed. Your husband is still waiting for you."

I got dressed, put back on my jewelry and walked out to the lobby. Walker was waiting on me. I felt fine. Bing Crosby was still ringing in my head....

DIAGNOSTIC MAMMOGRAMS CAN BE WRONG!

Dear Girlfriend,

After being told that I had breast cancer in the breast center by Dr. B, I received a letter dated December 10, 2008. The letter read, " We are pleased to inform you that the results of your recent mammogram are normal. A report of your mammogram was sent to: Doctor B." Girlfriend, I didn't know what to think. Can you imagine my confusion? Did I not have cancer? Was this whole thing just a big mistake? I wanted to just jump up and down for joy. I thought it was all just a big mistake! The diagnostic mammogram was normal. Yippee! I took the letter to Walker and he got really mad. "I can't believe they could make such a cruel error. Suzan, you do have cancer. Don't get excited. You do have cancer."

"Then why did they send me this letter? It says right here that a copy was sent to Dr. B. If the letter was wrong, why didn't he call me?"

"The only thing I can think of is that since you have such dense breast tissue, even the diagnostic mammogram just didn't show the lump. It's just outrageous that they sent a copy of this letter to Dr. B and he didn't call you to tell you it is a mistake. He knows you have cancer from the results of the core biopsy and the MRI. I'm really upset that they didn't call you to tell you it was a mistake. I think this is just another example of 'too many cooks spoil the broth'. His left hand doesn't know what his right hand is doing. If you choose to believe this letter, instead of the results of the core biopsy, then your cancer will just keep spreading and you know what that means..."

Girlfriend advice : If you feel a lump, the only way you can be posit-

ively sure that lump is not cancer is to have part or all of it removed!!! Do not ever depend or the results of a diagnostic mammogram or an ultrasound. They are sometimes WRONG!!! If you have dense breast tissue, that is breast tissue that still looks good, thick and rubbery, then lumps are often not detected, even by diagnostic mammograms!!! Get that lump taken out!!!

So after Walker read the letter I asked him, "What do you think we should do?" "I'm going to call Mac Molnar in Columbus. He'll know what we should do." Walker and I are both from Columbus, Georgia. Columbus is a hundred miles from Macon, Georgia, where we live, but we were ready to go any distance to find a doctor with whom we both felt comfortable. Mac is a lifelong friend of ours. He is an excellent surgeon and he would surely tell us what to do. So Walker called Mac and he recommended a wonderful surgeon named Dr. Ken Smith whose specialty was breast cancer. This doctor was a Fellow in Breast Surgery at Stanford University School of Medicine. Mac assured us that this doctor was the one to see.

So I wrote Dr. B a thank you note, and told him that I wanted to change doctors so I could have my surgery in Columbus, where my many relatives could give me lots of support. That of course was all true, but I didn't say anything about the letter fiasco. You are probably wondering why I was being such a wuss. Usually, I'm pretty feisty. Ask anybody who knows me! But when I was first diagnosed with cancer, I just could not deal with anything that was going to get me any more stressed out. I wasn't worried about Dr. A's slack nurse who didn't make my appointment at the breast center. I wasn't worried about Dr. B letting the inaccurate letter get to me. I didn't want any conflict in my life at that point. Like I said before, I was in survival mode. My only concern was to get hooked up with a doctor I felt comfortable with, a doctor who could save my life.

Christmas came. We did everything just like we had always done before. For Christmas dinner I bought some of those things that English people have at Christmas. They are called crackers. They look like the cardboard roll that toilet paper comes on, but they are wrapped in beautiful paper that is twisted on the ends. I put a cracker on everybody's plate. Before we started to eat we pulled the crackers open. They made a loud "CRACK!!!" sound that made us all jump. Inside each cracker was an extremely dorky tissue paper crown, an extremely corny joke printed on a small sheet of paper and an extremely tacky prize that looked like something out of a box of Cracker Jacks.

We all put on our crowns and took turns reading our jokes. The jokes were so stupid that we couldn't help but laugh. My oldest daughter, Laurel, was home from college. With her tissue paper crown on her head she read, "Where does Dracula keep his money?" We all shook our heads. "In the blood bank!" And so the day progressed with much merriment. I was the only one to touch the apple salad since all the girls said, "Bleck!!!" when I passed it to them. Olivia said, "Mama, why do you keep making this stuff? It's awful!"

"Awful? I love this stuff! I'm going to make it every year!" I replied.

So I made it through Christmas and on December 29, 2008, Walker and I headed to Columbus, Georgia to meet a fabulous surgeon named Dr. Ken Smith. I have many girlfriends, but the girl that has been my friend the longest is Suzanne. Suzanne and I became friends in 1970, our freshman year of high school. I was thirteen years old. This is now 2012, so we have been close friends for forty-two years. She was with me the first time I got drunk on sparkling Cold Duck. Ughhhh.... She was in my wedding. She gave me my first home permanent that made me look like Billy Crystal. She has been like a second mother to my girls. She is always there for me, so I was not surprised to see her sitting in Dr. Smith's waiting room when Walker and I came in the door. After filling out more forms, we were called back to the examination room. "Suzanne, do you want to wait? We could go to lunch after he's finished with me," I asked because I really wanted her to stay. "I'll wait for you. You look as white as a ghost," she said as I walked away.

Dr. Smith was middle aged with grayish hair and glasses. He was really nice. He was very business-like, but friendly and approachable. He smiled. Just that impressed me. After he had examined my breasts he led us back to his cozy office where I noticed that he had a bunch of pictures of his wife and family. I liked that too. He sat down with us and told us about all the different options I had for surgery. He drew pictures of what he would do if we went the route of a lumpectomy. " A lumpectomy only removes the tumor and a small amount of tissue around the tumor. I' ll do my best to keep your breast looking as much as possible like it does now. The pectoral muscles and lymph nodes will remain except for the first sentinel-node," he said.

"What is a sentinel- node?" I asked.

"The sentinel-node is the first lymph node that your cancer goes to if it has left the original tumor site. Before your surgery you will have a test where we inject blue dye into your breast. The dye will have radioactive particles in it. The lymph node that turns blue first is your sentinel-node. That is the node I will remove to see if cancer is in the node and from that I'll determine if we need to remove any more nodes, to see if the cancer has spread further. It could be that your cancer has not moved on to your lymph nodes at all. That's what we're hoping for."

I was starting to feel a little green around the gills. I didn't know much about cancer, but I did know that cancer travels throughout the body through the lymph system. I just kept thinking that my lump was so small that maybe the cancer had not gone on to the lymph nodes. Then Dr. Smith went on to explain statistics about breast cancer survival rates with and without chemotherapy. That's when I started to feel the room tilt a little. I sat in the chair and I could hear what he was saying. He was saying, " WAAA WAAA WAAA WAAAA... WAAAA... WAAAA... WAAAA........." I kept nodding my head like one of those little wobble head dogs that people put on their dashboards. I pretended that I was very interested in what he was saying, but inside my head I was trying my best NOT to hear what he was saying . I wanted him to just STOP TALKING!!!

I am here to tell you that it was a good thing Walker went with me to every single appointment the entire time I was doing the cancer thing. He went with me because he knew that if the doctor was saying something too painful for me to take in, I would just smile politely like I was listening, but in fact I would not be hearing anything but WAAAA...... WAAAAA...... WAAAAAAA........ WAAAAA........ WAAAAA..... WAAAAAAA..... WAAAA...... WAAAAAAA!!! My scared little wussy brain just could not handle survival statistics.

Girlfriend advice: Always take someone with you to every doctor's appointment who will listen to what the doctor is saying!

I know you think you are a big girl and can do this on your own, but why should you? Listen to me. Everybody knows you are a strong, intelligent, independent, modern woman. You have been diagnosed with cancer. Accept the help of your husband, lover, friend or relative. Believe me, if they are not really willing to go with you, to help you listen and digest what the doctor is saying, then they won't go. If they are willing to go with you, accept their help graciously. One day when you are well and strong you can return the favor. It really helps to have your helper take some notes. It has been my experience that what doctors think is just plain old everyday talk, can be pretty complicated and confusing to those of us who are hearing the cancer jargon for the first time. Also, let's face it, sometimes you might be so nervous that your brain just goes into the WAAAAA...... WAAAAA....... mode and your head just starts nodding and you may even hear your mouth saying, "Oh, I see...yes...I understand...." when you really don't see or understand anything at all!!! Understand?

Girlfriend advice: Don't dwell on survival rate statistics.

Dr. Smith was doing what he had to do. He was putting all his cards on the table. He was telling me all the routes we could take and to the best of his scientific knowledge, his statistics. He was telling me what my chances were to live for at least five years. He is an excellent doctor and I respect him immensely, but hearing those awful statistics scared me so badly that my brain refused to listen.

When we left his office, Walker, Suzanne and I went to lunch. Of course Suzanne said, "Well, what did he say?" I just sat there while Walker told her everything Dr. Smith said with a filter on it. He knew just what he could say without freaking me completely out. "Oh, he said that he is just going to take out that little lump. Her breast won't really look any different. It's going to be day surgery. She won't even have to stay overnight...."

"Oh, that's a relief! My God I've been so worried. Well, now I feel better. What are y'all gonna order. I'm starving...." Suzanne said as she read the menu.

"Walker, is that really what he said?"

"Pretty much. I took some notes about some stuff we can talk about later.... Let's just eat right now...."

So we made it through Christmas but New Year's Eve was harder. For the previous twelve years we had hosted a fantastic New Year's Eve party. Every year about one hundred and fifty friends and relatives would gather in the old house to help us bring in the new year. Some of our friends would come on the morning of the party, to help us blow up seven hundred helium balloons that we tied with multicolored shiny ribbon. We would let those balloons float up to the twelve foot high ceilings so that guests were walking and dancing through sparkly colored ribbons all night. It was really magical. There was always tons of food and a disc jockey to play music from Big Band to Rock and Roll. Everyone wore elaborate costumes. One year our theme was the roaring twenties. One year we had a Venetian masked ball. We started this party the year we bought the house, when it was still a dump. Nobody cared.

This party had become famous in Macon. I remember one year, a girlfriend of mine, Priscilla, insinuated that I was old. I said jokingly, "You better watch it. I'll take you off the party list." She of course apologized and begged me to keep her on the list. We had a good laugh, but before I put her invitation in the envelope, I ripped it in two. See, I told you I could be feisty. She called as soon as she received the invitation in the mail, "Oh, thank you so much for the invitation. I could tell by the condition it was in that I was walking on thin ice. And I just wanted to tell you that I have noticed lately how young and beautiful you are. You actually get better looking every time I see you!" I said, "Keep it up and you'll be safe." We both just howled, but from then on I'd always tear her invitation in two before I mailed it, just to keep her on her toes.

At the stroke of midnight back in 2000, a new millennium started with our house crammed full. There was barely room for me to crush through the crowd of revelers as I handed out bottles of champagne and party hats. The Disc Jockey led us all in the countdown, "Ten! Nine! Eight!...." The champagne corks were popping, the horns were blowing and everybody was kissing everybody.

Walker grabbed me as the whole crowd started singing, "Should old acquaintance be forgot and never called to mind...." We sang along as friends and family kissed us and hugged us.... We sang as loud as we could as our little girls pressed through the crowd to us. We held on to each other as the countdown ended and there was a deafening, "HAPPY NEW YEAR!!!" Walker kissed me long and hard .... We hugged our children as they blew their horns and we were all delightfully squished together by all our loved ones.

Then the D.J. cranked up, "When A Man Loves A Woman" by Percy Sledge, my absolute most favorite song. We danced and kissed and were kissed as we pushed our way out onto the front porch, where we discovered that the city was shooting off fireworks that could be seen clearly from our front yard. A first timer who had never been to a party at our house, thought we had arranged this tremendous fireworks display. He had on a hat made out of balloons, held a tasseled party horn in one hand and a half empty bottle of champagne in the other. He looked up at the beautiful fireworks as the music played, he put his arm around Walker's shoulder and said, "Fireworks! Man y'all thought of everything! When the Rivers throw a party they really throw a party!"

But on the night of December 31, 2008, there was no party. Even though we had finally finished the restoration of our home, we were not in the mood to have a party. I had just been diagnosed with cancer and we had spent every dime we could get our hands on to finish the work on the house. The only people at 923 High Street were the little Rivers family. One husband. One wife. Three daughters. We didn't know what to do with ourselves. The knowledge that I had cancer just hung in the air like something sticky and itchy. None of us knew what to say. Nobody wanted to say that they missed the party, but we all did. Nobody wanted to say that they missed the way things felt around our house before cancer floated under our door like a thick poisonous vapor to choke out our sense of peace and safety. We gathered in the kitchen around the table where we had always gathered every night as a family to say the blessing together and eat together. The phone rang. It was our friends Jack and Sterling. They called to say how much the party had meant to them and how they hoped everything would be better soon. Their call really meant a lot to me and I wondered if anybody else thought about what a hard night that was for us.

We played a board game as we sat around the table and just went to bed long before midnight. I heard the church bells down the street ring in the new year as Walker slept. I lay in the bed and wondered what was ahead of me in 2009. Thank God I couldn't see what was down the road....

LUMPECTOMY. YOU ARE BLUE. YOU LOOK LIKE A SMURF.

Dear Girlfriend,

On January 5, 2009, I started off the new year with a trip to my new medical oncologist. When you have cancer, there are so many doctors to keep up with. I had decided to let Dr. Smith in Columbus do the lumpectomy, but I had already set up an appointment with a medical oncologist in Macon before I decided to go to Columbus for surgery. Are you confused? Well, so was I. So far I had a primary care doctor and a gynecologist in Macon. I had a surgeon in Columbus and now I added a medical oncologist in Macon. The medical oncologist is the doctor who specializes in the treatment of cancer. Your surgeon takes the cancer out and your medical oncologist tries to keep it from coming back. The medical oncologist is the one who decides whether you need radiation therapy or chemotherapy to make sure the cancer does not return. Sometimes a cancer cannot be removed surgically, so it is the medical oncologist and possibly the radiation oncologist who work together to cure you without surgery. Whew!

I decided to go to the medical oncologist in Macon instead of getting a medical oncologist in Columbus, where my surgeon was, simply to save so much driving back and forth from Macon to Columbus. Bad mistake. Bad, bad mistake. This medical oncologist whom I will call "Doctor C", whose office was in Macon, had never laid eyes on my surgeon, Dr. Smith, whose office was in Columbus. This was not good.

Girlfriend advice: Try your very best to get a surgeon, a plastic sur-

geon, a medical oncologist and radiation oncologist who regularly work together, as a team, in the same town. If they don't even know each other and practice in different towns you may be setting yourself up for problems.

On my first visit to my new medical oncologist I should have seen red flags, but since I had no idea what to expect, I didn't see any. Walker and I entered Dr. C's office and filled out those same old forms, forms, forms. We sat down in the waiting room and I was called to have a nurse check my weight, pulse and blood pressure. She listened to my heart with a stethoscope and then I sat back down in the waiting room. Soon I was called back to meet Dr. C. Dr. C seemed very warm, however, Dr. C did not examine my breasts, which I thought was a little strange. Dr. C did not feel my lymph nodes in my neck or under my arms and did no blood work. In fact Dr. C never laid a hand on me, never examined me in any way, shape or form. Dr. C did tell me that if my surgery showed that cancer had moved to my lymph nodes, then I would need chemotherapy. Dr. C said that if cancer had not moved to my lymph nodes, a sophisticated genetics test would be done on the tumor, which might indicate that I had no need for chemotherapy. This test, called an Oncotype DX Test, is a tool used by oncologists to help them determine characteristics of the tumor, to help them choose the most effective course of treatment.

So we left Dr. C's office thinking that Dr. C would probably "do something" on our next visit. On January 12, 2009, I went to the hospital in Columbus for my pre-op. During this visit I went to the nuclear medicine office to be prepared for Dr. Smith to do the blue dye test, which would show the location of the sentinel node, during my surgery.

Walker and I have a cottage, way, way back in the woods on top of Pine Mountain, Georgia. Walker built this cottage himself with his good friend Gary Degler. This cottage is a stone Tudor cottage that looks like something out of Snow White and the Seven Dwarfs. "Fairy Ring Cottage" is just thirty minutes from Columbus, so we were able to sleep at the cottage on the nights before my appointments and surgeries and have a short trip to Columbus.

On the morning of January 13, 2009, we drove down the mountain to the hospital in Columbus for my surgery, which was to be on an outpatient basis. Can you imagine that you can have breast cancer surgery outpatient?

Well, you can, if you are having a lumpectomy. I arrived at the hospital and was taken back to surgery where I had to remove my clothes and jewelry and put on the lovely gown and a paper cap on my head. After that was done I was helped onto a gurney and an IV was started to help me relax. They covered me with a snuggy blanket that had just come out of a warmer. I was just laying there trying not to be scared when I was approached by a very talkative nurse. "Now, tell me what you are here for today, give me your name and date of birth," she said.

"I'm Suzan Rivers. My birthday is November1,1956. I'm here for a lumpectomy for cancer in my left breast." She nodded as she checked my plastic wrist band to make sure I was who the band said I was. Just as I was starting to feel the drug they had given me to relax she said, "Oh, honey, I had breast cancer too. First I had a lumpectomy and there was nothing to it. But let me tell you, that cancer came right back so fast and they had to do a mastectomy. Now that was awful...." I know my eyes must have gotten as big as saucers because she backed away as I said, "Can my husband come in now?"

"Sure honey, I'll go get him."

When Walker came back I was almost in tears. I told him what the nurse had said and he got so mad he said, "I can't believe anybody could be so stupid! Look, you are going to be just fine...." About that time Dr. Smith came in. We exchanged pleasantries, Walker kissed me and away they took me to the operating room. I only remember waking up. There was a nurse over me saying, "Sweetie, are you hurting? If you're hurting bad I'll give you some morphine. On a scale of one to ten, how bad are you hurting?" To tell you the truth, I wasn't hurting bad at all. I felt a little pain, but really and truly it wasn't bad at all. So I have no idea why I said, "Ten." That was all I said and the next thing I felt was WHOA NELLIE!!! She had given me morphine through my IV and I was for sure not feeling any pain.

Then I was taken back to the holding room where I had been before the surgery. Walker was with me. A nurse came by and said, "You can leave as soon as you go to the bathroom." Walker held on to my arm and helped me get up to go in the bathroom. When I came out he helped me put my clothes on. I asked, "Have you talked to Dr. Smith?" Walker said,

"Yes. He said it looked like he got it all. He only removed the lump, a little tissue around it and two lymph nodes. He said he didn't think that the nodes had any cancer, but we have to wait for the lab report to make sure. He sounded really pleased. I think you're going to be alright."

When I heard him say that I relaxed and that morphine really kicked in. As an orderly helped me get into a wheelchair and wheeled me out to the car, a tremendous feeling of well being settled over me. In the car on the way back to Macon I was as high as a hippie. I remember jabbering on and on about the morphine, "Wow! I can finally understand how people get hooked on this stuff. I feel great! I feel better than great, I feel incredible! I feel totally unafraid like everything is going to be alright! I feel...I feel... I feel like I'm going to throw up!" Walker pulled the car off the road and I threw up blue liquid. He looked at me and said,"Suzan, you are blue. I swear you look like a Smurf."

I got back in the car, and the nausea passed . I still felt high and happy. When we got back to Macon I made it in the house, but had to run to the bathroom to again throw up blue Smurf stuff. I had just finished throwing up and lay down on the beautiful new pink marble bathroom tiles when I heard my friend Priscilla's voice above me, "Are you okay?"

"I'm fine. Sorry I look so awful."

"You don't really look awful, but no kidding, you look blue."

I tried to laugh, but I really needed to get to bed. Walker and Priscilla and her daughter Coco helped me get upstairs to the bed. Soon the nausea passed and I really felt fine. My sister, Cea, was in town and she and Priscilla and Walker and Coco just stood around the bed talking and laughing about my looking like a Smurf. I was in no pain at all. If you are worried about a lumpectomy hurting, then you can stop worrying because your doctor can make sure you are not going to hurt. In a little while our neighbor Bill came over, "I can't believe you! You just had cancer surgery and you look fine. A little tint of blue, but you look great. You're talking and smiling like nothing happened. I can't believe this!" I really couldn't believe it myself. Other than a little vomiting caused by the anesthesia, I felt just fine.

Girlfriend advice: Don't fret over having a lumpectomy. It is not bad. If you talk to your doctor about pain control and nausea I'm sure he

can fix you right up.

With that first surgery, I remember that what stressed me out the most was my bandage. Dr. Smith had taped my breast up so tightly that it looked very flat. Walker kept telling me not to worry because Dr. Smith had told him that my breast was going to look almost exactly like it had looked before the surgery. But, every time I looked down, all I could see was flat on the left side. This really worried me. My surgery had been on a Tuesday. I rested in bed Tuesday, Wednesday and Thursday but not because I was in pain or even tired. I rested so that I would not forget that I had internal stitches that needed to heal.

Girlfriend advice: Even though you are not in pain, don't jump up for a couple of days because your stitches need a chance to heal. Remember you have internal stitches that you need to baby.

My surgery was on Tuesday and by Friday I was up hosting the Bible Gang. Lily said, "Look at you! You just had surgery. I can't believe it. You seem just fine."

"I feel fine," I said as we continued to eat chocolate cake and get caught up on the latest news. When all the "girls" except Mary had left, the phone rang. While still laughing at something Mary had said, as I answered the phone. "Hello, Suzan, this is Dr. Smith in Columbus. I got your pathology report and there was a little bit, a microscopic amount, of cancer in one of the nodes that I removed." I just sat down on the couch and immediately started to feel faint. "So what do we do now?" I asked.

"Well, I could go back in and take some more nodes to try to determine just how far it has gone. Since it was just a microscopic amount of cancer in the sentinel-node, there's a good chance that we already got it all."

"I want you to remove some more nodes just to make sure," I said.

"Okay, we can do that. I can do that outpatient. You are scheduled for your follow up appointment on the twenty-first. We can talk more then."

All I could manage to say was, "Okay." I hung up the phone and ran to Mary. I was so upset. "The cancer has spread to my lymph node. I have to have more surgery! Oh, Mary! I'm so scared! I don't want to die!"

Mary tried to calm me down, but this news had hit me like a thunderbolt. "Don't worry. We are all going to pray and everything will be fine…"

After she left I just went to bed. Once again I curled up in a little ball. Once again I pulled the covers over my head.... There was that old enemy, Fear, trying to put his hands around my throat again....

At my follow up appointment Doctor Smith removed my bandage and hey, you can't keep a good girl down. My breast popped right back up when he removed the bandage. The incision was like a very thin line around my nipple, even though the lump was down near the bottom of my breast. The stitches were all on the inside. The bottom of my breast, where the lump had been, had a very slight indention. All in all you could barely tell that I had had surgery. Dr. Smith had done a fantastic job. We set up the appointment for the second surgery to be on January 27, 2009. "When I go in to remove additional lymph nodes, I can go ahead and put in your port for chemo," Dr. Smith informed me.

"What is a port?" I asked.

"A port, or portacath, is something that you will be so glad you have while you do your chemotherapy. It's a tube that's inserted surgically into a vein in your chest. After it's inserted, the little hole where the tube ends will be stitched up. The opening to the port will be under your skin. Whenever you have chemo, or need blood drawn for any reason or need medications like antibiotics, the needle can be put into the port. That way you only have to deal with one stick, instead of having your nurse sticking you over and over again looking for a "good" vein. And the good thing is you can put a little Lidocaine on the skin covering the port to numb it, so that you don't feel anything when the needle is inserted."

I felt a little squeamish about the port, but it sounded better than a bunch of painful sticks with needles. I managed to say, "Okay." We left and went home to Macon. I felt like everything was starting all over again. Another surgery. Another gut wrenching period of waiting to see how far the cancer had spread. Then I got a call from my brother. He said my father was in bad shape and that I needed to come see him. Daddy was ninety years old. He and my mother separated when I was just seven. Daddy had been a pilot and a flight instructor in the Air Force. At the age of eighty-eight he went to live at an assisted living facility. Of course he wanted to keep his car. The problem was, that at that time, he had a stiff right leg. So he would hold on to the steering wheel with his left hand and lift his right leg with his right hand back and forth from the gas pedal to the brake pedal.

One night Walker and I were at dinner with some friends in Macon. I got a call from a nurse at the assisted living facility, "Mrs. Rivers, you have got to come do something about your father. He keeps chasing the nurses around in that motorized chair of his. He has this crazy idea in his head that he is in a brothel! He just chased one young nurse into the kitchen and she had to literally jump up on the counter to get away from him!"

"Yep! That's my daddy!"

So now daddy was dying, but what was he dying of? Not cancer. Not heart failure. He was dying from a pressure sore that he got from spending all his time in that motorized chair riding up and down the halls chasing nurses and anybody else who got in his way. What could have been more appropriate? He was a man who never stayed in one place. He had spent his life flying around the globe over and over, and he had spent his last few months flying up and down the halls of the assisted living home. Go daddy go!

He had been moved to my brother John's house in Atlanta his last few days and all six of his children were trying to get there to tell him goodbye. See, this is what I was telling you. When you are battling cancer you don't get to have any time out from life. Everything just keeps on going. You don't get excused from the hurt and pain of friends and relatives who will pass away while you are being treated for cancer.

But on the other hand, you don't get left out when somebody is telling a funny joke at a party. You get to hear it too. You get to laugh too. You can still hold a new born baby and smell that precious baby smell on the back of its little head. You can hold your daughter's hand while walking down the beach. You can watch your husband sleeping and think about how handsome he is even as he ages. You see, you are not left out of anything that happens to people in this life because you are still alive.

So Walker drove Laurel, Olivia, Blythe and me to my brother's house to see daddy one last time. When I walked in, all my siblings were laughing and talking and visiting in the kitchen just like nothing was going on. That's just what we humans do. We laugh to keep from crying. Daddy was at that age when he sometimes had his perfect right mind and sometimes he would just say things that were completely crazy. He had just told me a few weeks before he died that he had been communicating with different people in our family, some dead, some alive, on the VIN LINE. "It's the greatest thing! All I have to do is close my eyes and I can talk to you or Mama, [his mama died years ago] or anybody I want to talk to without a telephone!" I never tried to reason with him when he would talk about the VIN LINE because it would upset him. I would just go along with him and say, "Wow! That's so cool! I wish I could do that!"

That day, the last time I saw him, he was lying in bed, but he had his right mind. I just walked up to the bed and hugged him and held his hand. "You don't feel good?" I asked.

"Not so good. Are the girls with you?"

"Yeah, they'll come in to see you. You want to come see us in Macon?"

"You'll have to drive."

"That's fine. I can come get you in a week or two when you feel better." I said. Daddy had been baptized on his death bed just a couple of days before. He had managed to avoid being baptized for ninety years even though he had always believed in Jesus. "Daddy, I heard you were baptized."

He just looked at me and said, "Well, I figure it might not help, but then again, it couldn't hurt."

"No daddy, it sure couldn't hurt..." I smiled and squeezed his hand.

We didn't stay very long. When we got back in the car nobody said anything as we drove away. I started to cry and said, "I'll never see my daddy again...." No cancer doesn't give you any time out from life. No time out from being human. No time out at all....

Daddy died the day before my second cancer surgery which was on January 27, 2009. As I lay in the holding room on a gurney with my lovely little gown and paper cap on my head, my friend Mac, the surgeon who had recommended Dr. Smith, came by to see me. "Hey, Walker just told me about your dad. I'm so sorry."

"Yeah, I guess I won't get to go to the funeral."

"Well, you'll be out of here in just a few hours. Dr. Smith is a great surgeon. He'll take good care of you."

"I know. I really like him a lot." About that time Walker came back to kiss me goodbye once again. Dr. Smith came in and told me not to worry. That really meant a lot to me. Then I was off to the operating room again... I remember wondering how many times I would have to do this. Thank God we can't see too far down the road....Thank God we can't see too far down the road....

When it was over Walker was at my side telling me that Dr. Smith said he had taken out fourteen more lymph nodes from under my arm, and they all looked clear. "He seemed real happy. But you know the drill, we have to wait for the pathology report to come back," he said.

"You mean the scary pathology report..." I said as I tried to put the fear of the report out of my mind.

Girlfriend advice: Now remember what I told you. Make positively sure that you have signed the forms that will allow your doctor to talk to the person who is waiting for you to wake up from your surgery.

Your doctor is a busy man and he will scoot from doing your surgery right on to his next patient. If your husband is waiting to talk to your surgeon, he will be happy to talk to him, but only if you had your husband listed as the person to whom information should be released.

So we went home and the cards and flowers and books and visitors started pouring in. I am a member of The Intown Macon History Club, a small club that only allows fifteen members at a time. It is not that we are snobby, it's just that we wanted to meet once a month in a member's living room so we had to keep the group small. All of these women heard through that magical grapevine that I had cancer because I didn't try to keep it any secret. You would not believe the outpouring of love and prayers from these fifteen women.

I am also a member of a genealogical society. HOLY MOLY! I was inundated with so many cards that I just could not believe so many people out there cared so much about me. Girlfriend, surgery is great, but it is love that is going to heal you. The love of God and the love of your people will surround you and lift you to a place you have never been before. This place is the place where you actually realize how much you are loved. I know you know your husband loves you. I know you know your children love you. But did you know that woman down the street whose name you can't for the life of you remember loves you? You will get a card from her, a beautiful card, in which she tells you that she also had breast cancer, and she knows what you are going through, and she will put your name on the prayer list at her church. And you will think, " Why would she do that for me, I barely know her?"

Then you will start getting cards from women you have never seen before. The cards will say, "I know you don't know me, but your husband has done work for me. He told me about your trouble. I am so sorry. I had breast cancer twenty years ago. I am a survivor. You will be too!" And you will think, "Why is she sending me this card? I don't even know her. That is just incredible...." And the cards keep coming. Women that you know and women that you don't know send cards full of love and hope and prayers. "I am a forty year survivor." "I am a sixteen year survivor." "I am a twenty-two year survivor." "I am an eleven year survivor." And then you will feel literally lifted up.

You will be lifted up to a place you have never been lifted to before. You will know in your heart that you are a member of a sisterhood. This sisterhood of girlfriends, some have had cancer, some have never had cancer, but they have one thing in common. They honestly and truly do love you. And you will believe that, and that belief is what will get you through this mess that is cancer. I had a hard time thinking about those survival statistics that Dr. Smith had to share with me. I told my dear friend, Molly, about how those statistics were still haunting me. She said, "Suzan, those statistics left out one big factor- the healing power of love and prayer. People you don't even know are putting you on their prayer lists. You have literally thousands of people praying for you." What she said was true.

Thousands of people will pray for you, if you are open about having cancer. That knowledge will give you some strength. You will be like David facing Goliath. Instead of crying in your bed, all alone, so afraid of death that you can't begin to function, you will read those cards over and over and then you will pick up your slingshot, choose your rock, look that Goliath named Cancer in the face and say, "I will survive!!!"

The pathology report came back. All fourteen lymph nodes were clear. Walker and I went back to see my oncologist. Dr. C had read the pathology report, and reminded us that even though we had been told on our previous visit that if my cancer had lymph node involvement, I would have to go through chemotherapy, there might be a way to get out of doing chemotherapy. Since my cancer had only a microscopic amount of lymph node involvement in the sentinel node and the next fourteen nodes were clear, Dr. C said that there was some new research that had just come out about cases like mine. This new research said that if a patient had only a "micro- metastasis",which mine was, the tumor could still be sent to California for genetic testing. This test would tell us more about the characteristics of the tumor to guide further treatment.

This Oncotype DX test was extremely expensive, but what my insurance would not cover, Dr. C told us we could get paid by a private foundation. We went home and applied to the private foundation to pay for the genetics test, got approval, and Dr. C sent the tumor on its way to be tested. We waited and prayed.

When the test results came back to Dr. C, we returned to the doctor's office. As we sat in the waiting room the nurse called me over to check my pulse and blood pressure. The nurse told me that my heartbeat was irregular. That really surprised me because I had been to a heart doctor who told me that I had a rapid pulse, but not to worry because my pulse was not irregular. When I was called back I told Dr. C that the nurse said I had an irregular pulse. I asked Dr. C to listen to my heart. Dr. C listened to my heart and said that I did not have an irregular heartbeat. That was the only time Dr. C ever touched me.

Then Dr. C told us that the test on my breast tumor indicated that my tumor was extremely sensitive to estrogen. I thought of it like fertilizer. When my tumor was exposed to estrogen it grew faster. The doctor said that was actually the good kind of breast cancer to have because there are medications that keep estrogen from making breast cancer grow. Dr. C showed us the genetic test results that indicated that my tumor had only a ten per cent chance of recurrence. "So what does all this mean?" I asked.

"It means that I think you don't need to do chemotherapy," Dr. C answered. I looked Dr. C square in the face and I remember exactly what I said, "If these test results were your mother's, would you tell her not to do the chemotherapy?"

Dr. C looked me square in the face and said, "If these test results were my own I would not do chemo. Look, according to this test you have a ninety per cent chance that your cancer won't come back. If you do chemo that might raise your chances of no recurrence by about three per cent, but chemo is risky. You could have complications. You could get pneumonia. I don't think you should take all the risks of doing chemo when we have these test results saying you already have a ninety per cent chance that this tumor will not come back."

"So what do you think I should do?"

"I think we need to skip the chemotherapy, do some radiation treatments, and put you on a drug called Tamoxifen. Tamoxifen stops estrogen from hooking up with the cancer cells to make them grow. I think with Tamoxifen and radiation you will be fine."

I had never been so relieved in my life. I had been so afraid of chemo and now my doctor was telling me that I didn't need to do anything except take a pill once a day for five years and take some radiation treatments that wouldn't even make me sick. I was so happy! Dr. C also told me that I did not need to come back for a whole year. I didn't have to see Dr. C for twelve whole months because I was cured! Yippee!!!

Where were the red lights that should have been flashing? Why did I think it was okay to go without seeing an oncologist for twelve whole months right after having cancer surgery? Why didn't I think it was strange that Dr. C still did not even look at my surgery site to see what kind of job my surgeon had done? Dr. C never examined my breasts or checked my lymph nodes and never drew any blood to check my hormone levels. How could I have been so naïve? I wanted so much to believe Dr. C. How could I have been so stupid?

I went back to talk this plan over with my surgeon, Dr. Smith. He looked over the genetic tests results of the tumor while I told him that my oncologist had recommended radiation and Tamoxifen. He didn't act very enthusiastic about this plan. He didn't advise me against the plan, but I got the feeling that he was not enthused about my not doing chemotherapy. Now, if I had had a surgeon, an oncologist and a radiation oncologist who were all in the same town, they would have met together to talk over my case and plan their strategy together. That is the way it usually works. But, I had a surgeon a hundred miles away from my oncologist and they had never even met. Like I said before, I think I made a mistake picking out doctors that were in two different towns who didn't even know each other. I just didn't know any better.

"My oncologist recommended a team of radiation oncologists in Macon since the treatments will be every week day for a while," I told Dr. Smith. He said, "Alright, I'll set you up with an appointment to have your port removed, since you won't be doing chemo." He smiled and acted pleased, but I just sensed that he was hesitant about my not doing chemo.

The day I had surgery to have my port removed I went to a breast center in Columbus. I remember that I was not put completely out. I was in a sort of twilight sleep. The procedure was very fast. Surgery number three was no big deal at all. No pain. No nausea. No sweat. After the procedure I went with Walker over to my mother-in-law's house to rest for a couple of hours and then Walker and I met up with our surgeon friend, Mac, for lunch. Mac, as you recall, had recommended my surgeon, Dr. Smith.

I told Mac my good news about not needing chemotherapy. He smiled and acted pleased for me, but there again I got a funny vibe that he felt I should have gone ahead and done the chemo. Was this just my imagination?

When Walker and I got back in the car I said, " Did you get the feeling that Dr. Smith and Mac thought I should have gone ahead and done the chemo?"

"I don't know. Do you think you should do the chemo?"

"I don't know. I'm afraid of doing chemo, and I'm afraid of not doing chemo. I'm just afraid all the time. I'm just so sick of being afraid that the cancer will come back and kill me. I wish I could just have one day without fear. I think I've discovered that fear is the absolute worst feeling of all. I just don't want to be afraid anymore."

"Well, just get the radiation behind you and then see how you feel."

"Okay." I felt like all I ever said was "Okay." I knew so little about cancer that all I could do was trust my oncologist to be steering me in the right direction. I wish I had known then what I know now. Hindsight is twenty-twenty vision.

Girlfriend advice: If you go to an oncologist that does not ever examine your body or draw blood to check hormone levels etc. change doctors! You should be seen at least every three months your first year after surgery. If your oncologist puts you on a drug such as Tamoxifen, remember, there is a protocol the doctor should follow that includes seeing you at least every three months the first year.

RADIATION.

Dear Girlfriend,

Dr. C, my oncologist in Macon, recommended a group of radiation oncologists who were also in Macon. Walker went with me to the first appointment. We went in the office and once again filled out about a million forms. As I looked around the comfortable waiting room I realized that all those people had cancer. Nobody was freaking out. They were reading magazines and making small talk with one another. Nobody looked particularly afraid. I was afraid. I had been told by my oncologist that my cancer had a ninety per cent chance of not coming back, but I was still afraid. I was afraid that my cancer would come back. It just felt like I was getting off too easy....

I picked up a magazine. It was all about cancer. I put it back on the table and chose another magazine. It was all about cancer. Then I saw a cute little brochure with cartoon characters. It was all about the process of taking radiation treatments. I read through the little pamphlet about the way radiation was going to make me feel. It said that radiation would not make my hair fall out unless I was receiving radiation on my head. It is chemotherapy that causes breast cancer patients to lose their hair. The brochure said that radiation therapy might cause my skin to be "sunburned," but it said there were special lotions to deal with that. It said that radiation might cause me to feel fatigued. There was no mention of any very serious side effects to radiation. Yes, that's the part they left out...

I was called back to meet the doctor. He was going to prepare me to take external radiation. The radiation oncologist was very nice. When he first looked at my breast he said, "Where is your incision?" Dr. Smith had done such a good job during my lumpectomy that my little incision scar was hardly noticeable. My incision was around my nipple, but my tumor had been at the very bottom of my breast. Since it had been several weeks since my lumpectomy, the scar had almost faded away. I wondered how he was going to know just exactly where the tumor had been, since my incision was far from where the cancer had been.

He answered my questions. He told me that the possibility of radiation causing other cancers is very small, less than one per cent in ten years. "Why do I need this radiation if my tumor is completely gone?" I asked. "As far as we can tell you are cured, but there is always the chance that there is still a cancer cell in your breast that we need to kill. Radiation is just to raise your chances of not having a recurrence." Then he and the technician had me lie on a machine that took pictures of me from different angles. This is done so that the radiation will be administered in such a way as to not damage your ribs, heart and lungs. Measurements were taken of my breast. Then he marked my breast with ink. These ink spots were put on me so that the technician could direct the radiation to exactly the right spot each time.

I was so afraid of my cancer coming back that the radiation oncologist said, "Don't worry. It won't come back." I knew when he said that, that he was just trying to help me get over my fear of recurrence. He was just trying to be kind because no doctor can tell you for sure that your cancer will not come back. I was scheduled to start radiation on a Monday. I was supposed to come Monday through Friday at nine o'clock for twenty-eight days. I left the office afraid that even though I was doing radiation that my cancer would return.

Girlfriend advice: Listen to your inner voices. God has not spoken from a burning bush since Moses. God does speak to you when he puts very strong feelings of direction in you. Listen to your strong inner feelings and do what they tell you to do!

On Monday morning I went to the radiation center by myself. I didn't take Walker with me through my whole radiation treatment. When I was called back to do the treatment, I was given a cloth gown. I put on the gown and then went to sit in another waiting area until it was time for me to go into the room where the radiation was administered. There I was, wearing my little gown, sitting with three or four other little gowns. At least these gowns were not open in the back. I can't tell you how many times I have had to hold the back of my gown together, so I wouldn't be showing my mystery. By the time all of my cancer treatments were over, my "mystery" was not feeling very mysterious anymore!

So there I sat with the other gowns waiting for my name to be called. In front of me in plain view was a counter, and behind that counter was my doctor and several technicians looking at a screen. On that screen was the patient receiving radiation. The technicians reminded me of the Wizard of Oz, watching the screen while pushing buttons. When my name was called, a friendly technician took me over to the door of the radiation room. The door had a huge sign on it that said, "DANGER!!! RADIATION IN USE!!!" The door was made of metal and I swear it was about a foot thick. I just remember thinking, "I thought radiation was safe, but if I run out the door, this flimsy gown might fall off and I could be arrested for streaking!" I think that's why they put everybody in those gowns... so that they will have fewer escapees.

The technician escorted me into the radiation room and helped me lie on the table under the radiation machine. She helped me remove the top of the gown and positioned me exactly like she wanted me. Then she positioned the machine and said, "Now you just lie here and relax. I'm going to leave you alone a few minutes, but I'll be right outside watching you on my screen." I remember thinking, "Yep! You're scooting out because you read that sign on the door! What am I doing here? Didn't we learn in school that radiation is BAD for you???" I remembered back to when I was a little girl, we had drills at school, in case America was ever attacked with nuclear bombs. We children had to go and sit out in the hall, with our backs to the wall,while we held our geography books over our heads. I felt like yelling, "Hey! Y'all wait a minute!!! I don't have my geography book!!!" But before I had time to jump up and run out with her, that one foot thick metal door slowly closed automatically and the radiation machine started doing its thing. Yikes! It didn't really feel any different than getting any other kind of x-ray. It only took a few minutes before the tech was back in there with me, repositioning me for the next dose. All in all, I was only in the radiation room about fifteen minutes. I did not feel anything uncomfortable.

When it was over, the technician gave me a tube of cream and said, "Now, you need to apply this cream everyday, or your skin will start to look and feel sunburned. You're all done for today. Come back tomorrow at the same time." I said, "Okay...." and walked out of the office. I remember wondering how the radiation would affect me. And so it went, just like that for twenty-eight days of radiation.

For the first two weeks I really didn't feel any different, but as I went into the third week of treatment, I started to feel really tired. It was a peculiar kind of tired. It didn't make any difference if I slept more than usual, I still felt tired. I remember waking up in the morning feeling like I didn't have the strength to pull myself out of the bed, but once I did stand up and walk around a little bit, I felt okay. I made myself walk several blocks every day. That bit of exercise seemed to give me a little more energy. As the treatment progressed, my skin got a little pink from the radiation, so I just kept on applying the special lotion they had given me. I didn't think I was having any adverse reactions until months later, but then I really had trouble....

HE WAS JUMPING AROUND LIKE A MONKEY!

Dear Girlfriend,

My radiation treatments ended in June, 2009. I did not have an appointment scheduled with my oncologist until May 2010. My radiologists and my surgeon, Dr. Smith, kept up with me, but my oncologist did not. Dr. C didn't see any reason to see me that whole first year. So there I was with nobody drawing any blood, nobody checking my hormone levels, nobody checking to see if my cancer was indeed gone. That was the oncologist's job and Dr. C was not seeing me at all. Like I said before, I didn't think this was unusual because what did I know about oncological protocol? Zip! Nothing! I was just trusting my doctor's judgment and did not have a clue that that my doctor was not following proper protocol.

So the rest of 2009 went on by. I was going to go back to work as a school librarian, but discovered that my certification had expired .That meant that I had to go back to school to get a Master of Education in Library Media before I could go back to work. I enrolled at Georgia College and State University to work on my degree. My daughter was going to the same school and I can tell you it feels pretty weird going back to school in your fifties when everybody else is in their twenties! But this at least kept my mind occupied while I was adjusting to being "cancer free." Christmas rolled around and it was so much better than the year before because we all thought the cancer was gone.

On Christmas morning, I sat at the top of the stairs, while Walker went down to turn the lights on the tree. He hollered up the stairs, "Go back to bed girls! Santa Claus didn't come!" We once again knew he was lying and again ran downstairs together just like we had always done. I made the apple salad and again Olivia said, "Mama, this stuff is gross. It's worse than last year." I again replied, "This is real Waldorf salad. The recipe that they used at the Waldorf Astoria Hotel. It has to be good." And she again told me, "Mama this stuff stinks!" I again smiled as I dumped the salad in the trash....

We didn't have as much under the tree as usual because I was not working and the recession had really started to affect Walker's business. Nobody was buying timber because the housing market had crashed. When people are not building they are not buying lumber, and Walker is in the business of helping landowners sell their trees for lumber. Our business phone had practically stopped ringing. So now there was a new kind of stress in our home. Instead of worrying about cancer we were worried that we were going to lose the house. But hey, that is just the way of life.

The other thing that happened in 2009 that was very difficult for me was the deaths of five of my close girlfriends to cancer. All five of these women had been looking after me, trying to help me survive cancer, when they themselves were diagnosed with stage four cancers and within months all five of them were dead. Not only did I grieve at the passing of my friends, I grieved privately, because I didn't want my own daughters to see how sad I was. I felt like I just could not get to a place of real peace in my life. Fear of my own death was heightened by every funeral I attended. Another difficult situation that year was that my mother fell and broke her hip. So I moved into Fairy Ring Cottage for three months so that I could go to Columbus every day to check on my mother. At the same time I was driving back and forth to Macon to take classes for my degree in library media. I don't know how I managed all this while I was still experiencing radiation fatigue, but like I said, cancer doesn't give you any time out from life's other challenges.

If you think there is ever going to come a day when you will have all your eggs in one basket, and there is nothing difficult going on in your life, then think again. That day will never come in this life. This is the planet called Earth. On Earth you will never, ever reach the point of perfect happiness and perfect peace. If that is what you expect to achieve here then you might as will give up that notion. Here on Earth life is about constant challenges. You might be happy when you wake up, depressed by lunch time and in neutral by supper. Life is up and down, up and down, up and down. All you can do is grab onto every single minute of happiness you can find, when you find it, because it won't last long. You will never get to the point of constant, total happiness or peace in this life. If that is what you are expecting, then at the end of this life you will feel disappointed. This is not Heaven, the place of complete peace, this is Earth, the place where we must struggle constantly to be at peace that only lasts temporarily. We little Earthlings are at basic training, boot camp. If you expect anything different, if you can't roll with the daily punches life throws at you every day on Earth, then you will have a miserable life here.

So we did make it through Christmas again, and again New Year's Eve rolled around. We had no money to do the old party, so we took some family and friends to a great little restaurant and bar that is close to Fairy Ring Cottage, our little hide away house in the woods on Pine Mountain. Walker and I danced to country music and had just as much fun in bluejeans as we had ever had at our lavish parties in Macon. As he swirled me around the floor my mind floated back over the years....

When we first met in January of 1974, we were seniors in high school. When my mama and daddy met in 1938, they were in high school. That was the day of big band music. Every weekend my parents would go to a big pavilion in Columbus called The Idle Hour, where they would jitterbug the night away. Even though their relationship was rocky from day one, when he held her in his arms on a dance floor they had chemistry. They won dance contest after dance contest.

The whole time I was growing up all of my brothers and sisters loved to dance. We had a stereo in the living room. My sisters who were ten to fourteen years older than I, would turn on Chubby Checker and dance. When I was only five years old my sister took a home movie of me doing the peppermint twist. It was not unusual for one of my teenage sisters and her boyfriend to be slow dancing in the living room while I watched.

My mother always danced while she stirred gravy. Her hand holding the spoon would be going around while her shoulders and hips swayed to the music. I remember once in the 1960's after she and daddy had separated , she was just stirring that gravy while singing along with the radio to "I Can't Get No Satisfaction". So when Walker asked me to go to the prom in

1974, I expected him to dance. I was all dressed up in a red ironclad polyester formal . He had rented a tux with a ruffled shirt and had pulled his shoulder length hair back and tied it in a ponytail with a black velvet ribbon. We were styling! But when we got to the dance I was so disappointed that my handsome prince would not dance.

We married in 1976 when disco was all the rage. In the late seventies, John Travolta was busy ruining his back in "Saturday Night Fever." Wasn't he a hottie?! Walker and I at that time were living in Athens, Georgia, and going to the University of Georgia. To say we were living on a shoe string would be too generous. Let's say we were living on some scraggly little fuzz that hangs off a shoe string after its been in the tennis shoe about ten years. We were so broke Walker actually handmade our wedding invitations and delivered them on a bicycle to save the money for postage stamps. So, for us to actually go out to a disco was a big deal. Waitresses hated us because we would buy one beer and nurse it all night.

But, it was my birthday so we decided to go out. We went to a disco in downtown Athens that had a cover charge. After paying the cover we really only had money left for one drink. Now you have to remember that this was 1976. At that time in Athens, Georgia, black kids and white kids went to class together, but partied at different locations. Thank God we are past those days. So we paid our cover and when we got inside we realized that we were the only white people in the place. That didn't bother us and none of the black kids seemed to notice we were there, so we sat down and ordered our beers. When the waitress brought them Walker hollered in my ear over the loud music, "Drink it slow!" I longingly watched the other kids dance as he crumpled up little pieces of his napkin and put them in his ears. Everywhere there was sparkly light reflecting out of a large mirrored ball that hung over the dance floor. Walker and I just sat and sipped our beers and watched all those fellows in platform shoes get down.

There was a big long box about four feet high and twelve feet long out in the middle of the dance floor. It was covered in bright green shag carpet and had steps that you could walk up to be elevated so everyone could focus on the really good dancers up on this platform. "Wow!!! They can really dance!!! Look at their clothes!!!" I yelled in Walker's ear. "I'd rather die than get up on that thing!!!" he yelled back. "I'm going to the bathroom!!!" I hollered back and he nodded.

Now you know what the ladies room in a bar is like. All the girls have got a little buzz on and they all laugh and talk to each other even if they are total strangers. I told that to Walker once and he said, "Nobody talks in the men's room. We just do our doings and get out of there." But as I stood in line waiting for a stall to come open, a group of six rather rotund girls came in behind me. They were all laughing and talking and having a good time. One of them said, "How come y'all aren't dancing? Don't you like the music?" I said, "Oh, we love the music, but I can't get my husband to dance . He never dances with me." One of the girls that had a pretty major buzz, put her arm around my shoulder like we were long time friends. She started rocking her head from side to side and said ,"Girlfriend, we can sure fix that!" The other five girls all started laughing and giving each other the high five. "Honey, you just wait for us at the table, but don't you let on to your husband!"

So I just went back and sat down and sipped my drink. In a minute I saw the six girls headed straight for our table. They were laughing and giggling when the one I had talked to in the bathroom put her hand on Walker's shoulder and said, "Come dance with us!" Walker looked like he was about to faint as they all six pulled him up out of his chair and literally dragged him up the steps of the green shag carpeted platform. He turned and looked at me with the look of a condemned man being drug up the steps of a scaffold. I, of course, was enjoying every minute of this.

The six girls formed two lines and proceeded to bump Walker back and forth between them with their hips as the disco music blared out of the huge speakers so loudly that Walker stuck his fingers in his ears. He was as stiff as an old man with arthritis! He looked so pitiful until they all started pushing him back and forth amongst them while they were putting the bump and grind down on him. The D.J. started playing "Disco Inferno" by The Trammps. I was just cracking up! The music was blaring out so loudly that you could see the speakers vibrating. About that time I saw Walker was clapping his hands and jumping around like a monkey! He was bumping and jumping and winding and grinding while all six of those rather healthy looking girls worked him over real good. They had somehow flipped his switch! When the song was over he actually looked

74

disappointed as they took him by the hand and brought him back to our table. We were all laughing so hard we could hardly breathe. Then the ringleader of the girls put her hands on her hips, rocked her head from side to side, pushed Walker towards me and said, "Honey, we fixed him good!"

I owe an awful lot to those six girls because after that night Walker became a dancing fool. One time in the 1980's we went to a New Year's Eve party at the Columbus Country Club. I looked around and there was Walker doing the funky chicken with my brother-in-law. When Walker went back to work at the Georgia Forestry Commission on Monday, a man who had seen him dancing at the club told all the men that Walker supervised, "Boys, I hate to break it to you, but I saw your boss down at the Columbus Country Club dancing like a chicken with another man!" All the fellas said, "Boss man! Tell us it ain't so!"

I remember the last big New Year's Eve party we hosted . Walker was wearing what was supposed to be a toga but it came off looking more like Ebenezer Scrooge's nightgown. He had a wreath on his head made of gold laurel leaves. My nephew Todd and I were sitting together on the staircase as Walker was trying to jitterbug with my niece, Susan. He was pretty lit up and every time he twirled her around, he did it so fast and hard I was afraid he was going to throw her out the window. I said to Todd, "Now that is something I will remember the rest of my life." Todd just looked at me, shook his head and said, "That's too scary to think about!" See, I keep telling you these little flashbacks from my life so that you will believe me that cancer can't steal your memories. It can't steal your stories.

Girlfriend advice: Keep on dancing! Drag your husband into the living room, put on your favorite music and dance. When you are all alone at home and the fear of the future starts to overwhelm you, turn up your music as loud as you can and dance and dance until you drop. It will make you feel so much better. If you can hardly put one foot in front of the other from radiation or chemotherapy, when you feel your worst, start as slowly as you need to but do it! You won't believe how much better you will feel.

When we got back to the cottage long after midnight on that New Year's Eve of 2009, I felt so happy. I had such high hopes for 2010. I built a fire in my little fireplace and snuggled up in a soft blanket with my hot chocolate and I thought about how my life was going to be so much better than at had been in 2009. Thank God we can't see too far down the road....

RECURRENCE. LISTEN TO YOUR INNER VOICES.

Dear Girlfriend,

In January, 2010, I started a new semester of school, all of my classes were to bring my computer skills into this century. Woe is me. In the spring of 2010, I was assigned to do an internship in a public school library. I loved working with young children again, reading stories to them and doing puppet shows. Life seemed to be headed toward normalcy. I even planned to go back to work in the fall, but then the other shoe dropped. I have to tell you here and now that I have always had strong inner feelings that I allow to guide my actions. So in the spring of 2010, right when every thing in my life was at last starting to settle down a little bit, I started having strong feelings that my cancer might be back. At first I tried to ignore these feelings, but they just would not go away. At night I would lie in bed reading a book while Walker slept away peacefully beside me, but I couldn't concentrate on what I was reading. I just kept having this overwhelming feeling that something once again was wrong with me.

"Suzan, you've got to get past this. God let you live! Look at all your friends that died of cancer last year. You've been given this great gift of life. You've got to stop being scared and start living! Enjoy this life you have, stop ruining it with all this worrying! You have just got to put your cancer behind you and live!!!" Walker said this over and over but every night the same thing would happen. I would choose the lightest and happiest books I could find to read to keep my mind off the feeling that my cancer was back. I read the Mitford series. I read James Herriot. I read tawdry romances, anything to drown the dark feelings inside of me, but nothing seemed to help.

"Walker, I'm going to go back to the radiation oncologists. I'm going to tell them that I want an MRI. I just can't stop having this feeling that something is wrong with me," I said. " Okay, but at this point your insurance has run out. You were able to stay on Cobra since you quit working, but now that has run out. You might have a hard time finding more insurance because you've had cancer," he replied.

You can't imagine how hard this hit me. I had never up until that point thought of myself as so seriously sick that I was a high risk person as far as insurance companies were concerned. I really wanted that MRI, but an MRI would cost about $3600 and with myself and three girls in college, not to mention Walker's business was going steadily down, I just did not have an extra $3600 to pay for the MRI. This was the first time in my life that I was uninsured, so I was even afraid to drive to the grocery store for fear that if I was injured in a car wreck, I would not have money for medical care.

I went ahead and made an appointment with the radiation oncologists. This time I saw a different doctor. He was very young and very handsome. He had a warm and caring personality. After he examined my breasts I said, "I keep having these ominous feelings that something is wrong, and that I should have an MRI to get it checked out." "Suzan, your Oncotype DX test indicated that you only have a ten per cent chance of a recurrence. You're fine. You need to just relax and enjoy your life. Enjoy being cancer free. Embrace your wellness!" I wanted more than anything in this world to just take his advice, leave cancer behind and go live my life, but I just couldn't do it.

"I want to embrace wellness, but there is a feeling deep inside of me that's telling me to get an MRI. Something is wrong with me and I think it might be God who's putting these strong feelings in me. Hasn't anybody else told you something like this before?" I asked. He stopped talking and said, "Yes. I've heard other people say that they're having strong feelings that are telling them to do this or that, and I'll have to admit that most of the time the feelings are telling them to make the choice that turns out to be the right thing to do. I'll order you an MRI," he said. "Well, there is just one little problem. My insurance with Cobra has run out and I don't have $3600 to pay for the MRI," I answered. He just looked at me a minute and said, "I have an idea. I'll call the insurance commissioner for the state of Georgia and maybe he can tell us a way to get you some insurance. With your good prognosis and the fact that you are willing to pay for the insurance on an individual plan, maybe he can do something." "I can't tell you how much I appreciate this," I said as I left his office.

I went home and told Walker what the doctor had said. "You know I've been talking to the insurance commissioner's office myself," he said. "I would have never in a million years thought of talking to the state insurance commissioner's office. I think that it's no coincidence that you and my radiation oncologist were thinking the same thing. You know the Lord works in mysterious ways. Maybe He's telling me that I need to have that MRI and He's showing you and my doctor how to make it happen," I said over my coffee cup. "Suzan, I've learned to pay attention when you get these inner feelings," Walker said.

"Well, I don't take any credit for it. I think God puts feelings of guidance in everybody, but maybe I've just trained myself to listen to these feelings more than some other people do. In the quiet, after you're asleep, when the house has settled down, I just listen to my feelings. I don't hear any voices like Moses did, just persistent feelings that tell me what to do."

As it turned out, I could get insurance. The state of Georgia makes their insurance companies take a certain number of customers, whose Cobra insurance has previously run out. So, I was assigned to a particular insurance company and even though my cost is expensive, most of my medical bills have been paid by my insurance.

I went back to the MRI center and went through the same test all over again. The results were sent back to my radiation oncologist. A few days later he called me and said, "Suzan, I got the results back from your MRI and there is a suspicious area close to where you had the lumpectomy. I think I'll send these results to your surgeon." I thought I would die. "Okay. Thanks for letting me know," was all I could manage to say. In a few days time my surgeon, Dr. Smith called, "I really don't think you have anything to worry about. I believe what we are seeing is just scar tissue, but we can do a biopsy just to make sure."

"Okay," was again all I could manage to say. This would be surgery number four. I could not believe my ears. I was going to have surgery again. I was going to have to suffer through waiting for the results of that surgery again. When the day arrived for me to have the surgery, Dr. Smith came to see me before I went in for the operation. "I really don't think there is anymore cancer, but just so you won't be worried, I've arranged for a radiologist to do an ultrasound on that area that looks suspicious on the MRI. She'll be able to tell us what she thinks before we go in to do the surgery." Once again I managed to say, "Okay."

The radiologist did an ultrasound and said, "I don't see anything that looks like cancer. I think you can go into this surgery without worrying." What she said made Dr. Smith and me very happy. Once again I was put to sleep as Dr. Smith removed the suspicious area. When I woke up from that surgery, I was able to go on home feeling confident that everything was going to be alright. Thank God we can't see too far down the road.... If I had known what lay ahead of me, I don't think I could have made it through.

Several days passed. I was sitting at the kitchen table with my daughter Blythe when Walker came in the kitchen. He was crying. "Oh, I just talked to Dr. Smith, you have cancer again!" I jumped up from the table and burst out crying, "I was right! I kept telling you it was back! I'm going to die!" Walker grabbed me and held me tight. We both just stood there holding on to each other crying and crying. Then I realized that my precious daughter was seeing us fall apart for the first time. Oh, there had been plenty of falling apart on the first go around, but not in front of her. That was the first time she had seen her mama and daddy just fall apart right in front of her. I felt so bad that I had lost it that I just pushed Walker away and ran upstairs.

Once again I went to my bed, and once again I pulled the covers over my head. In a minute I felt Walker crawl into bed behind me. He wrapped his big strong woodsman arms around me while we both cried. What else could we do? I felt my tears drip down his arm and I wiped my face with the bed sheet. "Oh, Walker, I can't do this again! God, I can't go through this again! They're going to cut my breasts off this time! I can't do this!" I cried and cried until I had smeared mascara all over my face and my nose was running all over Walker's shirt. Then I thought about the children I had seen in the hospital who had cancer. These precious little children were bald and wrapped up with blankets. They were holding on to their teddy bears and stuffed bunny rabbits while nurses pulled them to radiation in those old-timey red Radio Flyer wagons. None of them were crying. I felt ashamed. I got up and washed my face....

OFF WITH MY OLD BREASTS AND ON WITH THE NEW.

Dear Girlfriend,

After I was told that the cancer was back, I went to see my surgeon, Dr. Smith. I think he felt badly because he had been so confident that the cancer had not come back. I sat on the examination table in his office trying to hold it together as he broke the news to me, "I think this time we should remove that breast." I just could not believe this nightmare was happening to me. "Everything I've been told was wrong! Everybody was sure it was gone and now you're telling me I need a mastectomy. What about the other breast?" I asked. "Well, sometimes women opt to just go ahead and take the other one, too, so they don't have to spend their lives wondering if the other one will have cancer. Is that what you want to do?"

"Yes. I just can't stand the thought of going through all this again."

"Well, one good thing about having them both off is that you have a much better chance of their matching if you do reconstruction. You can even have new nipples made, but they won't have any sensual feeling like real nipples," he said.

"Then that's what I want you to do. Just take them both."

"Okay. We'll get approval from your insurance to have another port for chemotherapy put in, a bilateral mastectomy and reconstruction. Do you have a plastic surgeon here in Columbus?"

"Mac Molnar recommended Dr. Vince Naman. Do you know him?"

"Yes. We work together all the time. We may be able to remove your breasts and put in your implants while you are still under anesthesia. That way when you wake up everything will be done and you won't have to be put under anesthesia again for another surgery. You go to sleep with the breasts you have now and wake up with new breasts. You won't have nipples, but those can be done later. This way you won't have the trauma of waking up with no breasts," he said. I liked the idea of going out with my old breasts and just waking up with new ones. The trauma of waking up with no breasts was just more than I could handle at that time.

So, the next step was to go and meet Dr. Naman. What can I say about Dr. Naman? Dr. Vince Naman is a graduate of Princeton University. He earned a fellowship to the Mayo Clinic in Rochester, Minnesota, where he completed his training in plastic surgery. I first met Dr. Naman in May of 2010. It is now November, 2012. This means that I have known Dr. Naman and his staff about two and a half years. I feel like I have known them my whole life. They have been so incredibly good to me. If it were not for their medical expertise and their caring attitude, I don't think I could have made it this far. I remember the first time I went to Dr. Naman's office. I was terrified. I was afraid of having my breasts removed. I was afraid of chemo making me sick. I was afraid of losing my hair. But above all else, I was afraid of dying. I had just seen five of my friends die of cancer. I had been told just one year before that I was "cured," and now the trauma of being told that the cancer was back was almost more than I could bear. I was taking something for depression and anxiety which made it possible for me to function during the day, but at night, when everyone else was asleep, a blanket of fear did its best to smother me. I once again felt like an axe murderer was chasing me around my house and I had no where to run and nowhere to hide.

That was the shape I was in the first time I walked into Dr. Naman's office. After I had filled out all the forms, Debbie escorted me back to an examination room, where I put on a cloth bib that covered up my breasts and my back. It was open on the sides. I know you are probably wondering why I bothered to tell you about this cloth bib, but after you have had so many people looking at your bare body, you learn to appreciate that somebody is thoughtful enough to give you a cover up that will actually hide your nakedness. I appreciated that I could talk to Dr. Naman without feeling like a chicken that had just been plucked. This might sound like no big deal to you, but I have come to appreciate little things like a modest cover up as a sign of caring and respect.

After I put on the bib, Debbie gave me a brag book to look through. She left the room and Walker and I sat and looked at actual before- and -after photographs of women who had had bilateral mastectomies. Of course these photographs were of the breast area only. Looking back on it, I remember that I was disturbed by the scars on the breasts. Now I realize that those pictures must have been made shortly after surgery. For the most part the scars do fade. Until they do fade, you can apply a cream makeup on the scars and they are almost invisible. I do not remember seeing any pictures of what a woman looked like with no breast, I mean before the implant was put in her. Now, I wish I had asked to see some of those photos.

When Dr. Naman came into the room he was friendly and upbeat, but to tell you the truth I felt like a three-ring circus could not have put me in a good mood at that point. I was afraid and I was embarrassed to have another man that I did not know look at my breasts. After we had exchanged pleasantries, I told him that I wanted my surgeon, Dr. Ken Smith, and him to work together. I wanted to be put to sleep with my old breasts and wake up with new ones. Dr Naman told me that he would be willing to do that, but he warned me that many times women who have had a radiated breast have trouble doing reconstruction after a mastectomy. This was the first time I had ever heard this. My radiation oncologists never mentioned that radiation could make my skin so weak that it could not hold an implant. "Sometimes the skin is so damaged by radiation that the implant tears out," Dr. Naman told me. I was flabbergasted that my radiation oncologists had not warned me of that problem. They had only told me about my skin feeling "sunburned."

I suppose they did not mention this to me because they thought I was cured and that all my surgery was over. I suppose they thought there was no reason to mention that radiation can cause the skin to be thin and weak like a wet paper towel so it just can't hold in an implant. "A lot of times I do what is called a latissimus dorsi muscle flap surgery. I think that's what I should do with you," he said.

"What is a latissimus dorsi muscle flap surgery?" I asked. "That's when we take tissue from your back, from the latissimus dorsi muscle, leaving the skin and the artery attached, and push it from your back around to the front, under your skin. This new strong skin taken from your back will replace the old radiated skin that might be too weak to hold your implant. The muscle we use to help build the breast mound, but most of the time we put an implant under the muscle. A silicone implant feels more natural than saline most of the time."

"What about the scar on my back?"

"The scar on your back will be a slightly curved thin line about ten inches long."

Together we looked at the book of photographs and they looked pretty good. Then I saw one photograph of a woman whose breast was not exactly in line with the other one. This picture bothered me and I said, "What happened to this lady? Her breasts are sort of lopsided." Dr. Naman looked at me with a straight face and said, "Oh, I just didn't like her so I did that on purpose." I must have had a horrified look on my face because he said, "I'm just kidding! This lady had breast cancer that was a lot more advanced than yours. That was just the best we could do, but she was actually very happy with the results." For the first time I relaxed. I realized that he had a fun personality to joke about how he just didn't like the lady so he made her lopsided on purpose. I remember I actually smiled and said, "Well, I certainly hope you like me because I don't want mine to be lopsided!" Walker, Dr. Naman, and I all laughed together for the first time and I started to feel a lot better about the surgery. When we left his office, I had the feeling that he was extremely competent and had a good, fun, and caring personality that had put me at ease.

Finally, I had a good cancer surgeon and a good plastic surgeon, but I didn't want to stay with the oncologist who had totally ignored me for the entire first year after my lumpectomy. I had done some research and found out that there was an entire protocol that Dr. C was supposed to follow after putting me on Tamoxifen. My oncologist had not followed any protocol. Dr. C completely ignored me while my cancer came back. I went to my friend, Mac Molnar, and asked him to recommend an oncologist. Mac recommended Dr. Andy Pippas at the John B. Amos Cancer Center in Columbus, Georgia.

So there I was, off to meet yet another doctor, hoping and praying that this doctor would actually take care of me and care about me. The day I met Dr. Pippas, I was just as scared as I was on the day I met Dr. Naman. Dr. Pippas completed his residency in internal medicine and a fellowship in medical oncology/hematology at Duke University Medical Center in Durham, North Carolina. Dr. Pippas is an incredibly wonderful oncologist, but his personality is very serious. He doesn't smile very much and that made me very nervous because I love to laugh and joke around. Even through battling cancer I tried to look on the light side. The first thing he asked me was, "Why are you wanting to change doctors?" I said, "I went to an oncologist who never examined me, never touched my body one time except to listen to my heartbeat. At my request. All Dr. C did was send my tumor off for an Oncotype DX test. It was determined through this test that my cancer only had a ten per cent chance of returning, so my oncologist just turned me over to the radiation oncologists, gave me a prescription for Tamoxifen and said for me to come back in a year. The only way I knew that my cancer had returned was from my own ominous feelings. I just knew, God told me that my cancer was back." Dr. Pippas didn't comment on what I said, but he did accept me as a patient.

From that very first day he ran every kind of test that was appropriate to determine my white cell count, my hormone levels etc. etc. He was so thorough that I felt so taken care of, which was a totally new feeling for me. He didn't smile very much, which was really scary for me. When a doctor smiles it makes me feel like everything is going to be alright. But, even though Dr. Pippas didn't smile much, he was a fantastic doctor, because he listened to me and took my every complaint about my body seriously. If you need a good oncologist I can highly recommend Dr. Andrew Pippas.

Dr. Pippas had a Nurse Navigator named Lori. A nurse navigator runs interference between the patient and the doctor. Dr. Pippas is such a busy man that he can't take every call that he gets from his many patients. Lori would take my calls, talk to Dr. Pippas and then promptly call me back. Lori always looked like she was running a marathon and whatever she was paid should have been doubled. She was the one that dealt with an incredible amount of patient stress, strain, fear and downright hassle. I don't know how she did all that she did, but hopefully you will choose an oncologist who has a nurse navigator just like her. Everything ran so much more smoothly because of Lori. She deserved a medal.

So, a few days later, it was time for the big show. This was surgery number five. I entered the hospital in the morning and they put me in the lovely gown with the matching bonnet. I was put on a gurney and an IV was placed in my arm. They started giving me some good dope in my IV to calm me down because I was so scared. Walker was able to stay with me in the holding room, and that helped to relax me. In a little while Dr. Naman came in and sat down on one of those rolling stools that he pushed up next to my gurney. That made him face to face with me, and he talked very sweetly to me. Now, you probably wonder why I tell you little details like, "That made him face to face with me." Well, let me tell you, when you are about to be rolled down the hall to have both of your breasts amputated, any little gesture of kindness you will remember for the rest of your life. Just having him talk to me eye to eye was so much more personal and made me feel so much more cared for than if he was standing up tall, looming over me.

He said, "Listen, if you want me to, I can forget the latissimus flap surgery and just let Dr. Smith remove your inner breast tissue and save the radiated skin. Then I can just slip a saline implant in and that's a lot less involved than the flap surgery." "Well, you said you were worried that since that left breast was radiated, that it might not be strong enough to hold the implant," I said. "You have about a fifty-fifty chance that it will hold. Do you want to give it a try? We might get lucky. And I think I might have a better chance of getting your breasts to match if I use saline instead of silicone." I said, "Let's give it a try and if the implant holds I won't have to go through such a big surgery." "Okay. We'll just say a prayer that everything turns out alright." He took my hands and bowed his head and asked God to take care of me through the surgery. Dr. Smith came in and said, "Okay, I think we're ready to roll!" Walker kissed me goodbye and off I went to surgery.

I never really understood before just exactly how a breast is removed. In most cases they are able to save your skin. So think about a cantaloupe that has been cut in two. That half cantaloupe is your breast. They just scoop out the inside of the cantaloupe and leave the rind. So think of your breast . An incision is sometimes made across the breast so that the breast can be opened up and the tissue right up to your skin is removed. I asked Dr. Naman if he could cut my breast around the bottom so the scar would be less visible. That is what he did on the breast that had not been radiated. You will also have an incision to remove your nipple. The thought of not having nipples when I woke up from surgery was really creeping me out. But, I had to just keep saying over and over in my head, "This is only temporary. This is only temporary." That's what you will have to keep saying to yourself in order to get through your treatment.

There is something else I want to tell you. When you hear the words "you need a mastectomy," just remember that what is going to be removed is your internal tissue. That tissue will be replaced with an implant. So what you have always seen your whole life, your skin, will still be there. Of course if you have to do a latissimus flap surgery your breast will be partially constructed with skin from your back, but that is still part of your body, it's not fake, it's real. Some women opt for the tissue to build a breast to come out of their abdomen. This method can actually allow the doctor to give you a tummy tuck in the process. But, what I'm trying to say is that when all is said and done, what you see is not fake. It is your skin, taken from your body.

So don't think of your breasts as "fake", they are made out of your skin and sometimes are partially built with your own tissue. Yes, even the center part of your nipple, the part that stands out when you are cold, can be reconstructed with your own breast skin or tissue taken from other parts of your body such as your inner thigh or ear lobes. The areola, the colored part of your nipple, will be made by tatooing your skin. You can help picking out the color. That reminds me of looking at paint samples. So, unless you for some reason need to have an artificial implant in the center of your nipple, other than your tattoos, your breasts are "real". Everything that you see on the outside is real skin taken from your own body. Of course you won't be able to breast feed a baby again, but you will be able to show off your own real skin in a low cut dress or bathing suit. This will help you to feel pretty and sexy again.

I had to keep reminding myself that I was lucky. What if I were having a leg amputated? Then I remembered my cousin, Ken. Ken had a melanoma on his nose that was so bad that he had to have his entire nose removed. Can you imagine the nightmare of having nothing but a gaping hole where your nose has been? Ken told me, "I was in the hospital room with another man that had the same exact surgery. That man would not go out of his house for all the months and months it took to do his nose reconstruction. I thought that if I let my surgery keep me from going on with my life, then it would be like letting Cancer win. I wasn't about to let Cancer win. The doctor showed me how to bandage my face. Nobody knew what was under that bandage but me. When I went to the grocery store or the movies nobody even batted an eye at me. Nobody freaked out because I had a bandage on my face. I just kept on going just like nothing ever happened." I thought that if Ken could go through the horror of having his nose completely removed, then I could go through having my breasts removed. His testimony about his experience really helped me a lot. Until I got the morphine....

It was a seven hour surgery. My breasts were opened up for a very long time. Anytime your body is opened up for so long you are at risk of getting a staph infection inside your body. But, I was willing to take that risk because I was so afraid of waking up with no breasts. When I finally did wake up, I started to cry. I was taken to my room, but I just could not stop crying. I was in no pain at all, so you don't have to worry about that, but I could not stop sobbing. Dr. Smith and Dr. Naman both came to the room and held my hands and tried to comfort me, but I could not stop crying. I was crying for two reasons. First of all, I was terrified of the pathology report. I was afraid that they were going to tell me that the cancer had spread and I didn't have a good shot at living. The second reason I was crying was because I was on a bad morphine trip....

EVERYBODY HAS TWO HEADS!

Dear Girlfriend,

When I had the lumpectomy the year before, they must have given me just enough morphine to take away the pain and give me an extremely pleasant buzz. This time I was on a bad trip and it was scaring me to death. Every time I looked at somebody for more than a few seconds they would form a second head. I don't care how attractive a person might be with one head, they are down right scary looking when they have two. So I was terrified to look at anybody and I just kept on sobbing. And to add insult to injury they had put my legs in those squeezy leggings. These leggings would inflate with air and then deflate to keep my circulation going so I wouldn't get a blood clot. But, the problem was they made my legs and feet itch. So there I was afraid of the path report, afraid to look at anybody because they all had two heads, and my legs were itching like fire inside the squeezy boots. Walker's nickname for me is "Boo Boo". I remember him just shaking his two heads and saying, "Poor little Boo Boo...."

Since this crying jag continued all through the night, Dr. Smith asked a psychologist to come talk to me. It just so happened that when he walked into my room, without even knocking, the nurses had just, for the first time, gotten me out of bed and put me on a potty chair. So there I was on the potty with my lovely gown wide open in the back, once again exposing my mystery, when in comes this psychologist. Without even introducing himself he launched into why I needed to stop crying. Now you have to remember that I didn't know this jackass from Adam's house cat, but I allowed him to wax poetic for a few minutes until I finally asked, "Who are you???!!!" "Oh, I'm Dr. I (I stands for idiot!) I'm a psychologist. Dr. Smith was concerned about your being so distraught, so I have come by to talk to you." "Well, did you just happen to notice that I am naked and sitting on the potty? I can't talk to you. Please leave!"

Can you believe that? How can you talk about your psychological problems sitting on the potty? I was just blown away. The next morning this dingbat came back again. This time he brought a female intern with him. I suppose he had planned to show her how to get an overwrought woman to calm down. This time I was in the bed but those squeezy leggings were making me itch so badly that I was about to go nuts. I was taking my foot and rubbing my other foot under the covers to try to stop the itching. Dr. I just sashays in again and this time says, "You know, you really just need to get this cancer under control." At that I switched off feet and was really going at the scratching under the covers. Then he said, "I can tell that what I just said really had great impact on you because I can see you are swinging your crossed legs under the covers."

I guess he thought that what he had just said must have really impressed the female intern because he turned and gave her a very sage look as he crossed his arms over his chest. I said, "What you said had no effect on me. I just have itchy feet!" At that the intern giggled a little which I guess hurt his pride, so he repeated, "I said that I think you need to get this cancer under control." I just looked at Walker and he had seen that look in my eyes before. He knew I was about to take Dr. Idiot out. Now, normally I am a warm and loving person, but this Bozo had just gotten on my last good nerve. I pushed myself up in the bed and said, "Do you think that I can control my cell division? Look at that bald head of yours, can you make your hair grow back???!!!" At this point the female intern actually started laughing out loud.

Then I said, "Having cancer is about realizing that you don't have control. Yeah, I can eat right and not smoke or drink. I can do everything just exactly right, but I know that this cancer can still come back and kill me. Control? Having cancer is all about realizing that human beings have pretty much no control over their bodies. Can you control your heartbeat? Can you control the inner workings of any organ inside of your body? You can't do any of those things. You're on automatic. Everything in your body is working and doing what it needs to do because the power of God is keeping you running. Having cancer brings you to that realization. The realization that no matter what you do, one day your body will die because that is just the way God allows it to be and there is not one thing you can do about it! Having cancer brings you face to face with the fact that ultimately God is in control of your body, not you! Cancer is about accepting the knowledge that God is in control, and you just have to trust that when you do die, He'll continue to be in control, and take care of you on the next stage of life after this one!"

Well, let's just say he drew back a nub. The intern nodded her head and smiled and Dr. I just took his two big bald heads and left. Walker said, "Well, I don't think he'll be coming back." I just lay back down and said, "I hope not," and went back to scratching my feet and crying. A couple of hours later a very nice gentleman knocked on the door and said he was a psychiatrist. I guess they were sending in the big guns since I had shot down the little bald-headed gun. The psychiatrist was very friendly and asked me what I had said to Dr. I. I told him pretty much word for word what I had said. The psychiatrist said, "That's about the most sane thing I've heard anybody say in a long time. I think when you get a good path report back and they can get you off this morphine, you will feel so much better. If you want me to come back just call me. If not that's okay," I thanked him and he left.

Shortly after that Dr. Naman came by and told me the path report was great. They found absolutely no more cancer in my left breast. Dr. Smith had gotten it all out when he did the initial biopsy at the breast center. As it turned out, my other breast did have some precancerous cells in it, so I had made the right decision to have it removed. Dr. Naman then took me off the morphine and everybody went back to having just one head. He put me on some mild painkillers so I actually had no pain through the whole experience. The crying stopped, the itching stopped, and after thirty hours I finally fell asleep....

Girlfriend advice: Ask your doctor to get the pathology report back to you as soon as possible after your surgery. Make sure your support person is there with you when your doctor brings you the report. Find out what painkiller your doctor plans to use and see if you will possibly experience hallucinations. If so, see if there is something else he can use. Also, if you have unbearable itching, you may be allergic to opiates. Morphine, Demerol, Hydrocodone and other pain medicines are derived from opium. If you wake up from surgery with unbearable itching in the area of your surgery or if you are itching from head to toe, ask your doctor about using a painkiller that is not an opiate. If it is just the squeezy leggings that make you itch, you can use a topical skin calming lotion such as Sarna daily to help ease the itching. In my book itching is worse than hurting.

UNVEILING THE NEW BREASTS. NOT BAD AT ALL!

Dear Girlfriend,

The next day while my friend Suzanne was there with me, Dr. Naman came by to change the bandage. Walker was there, too, but I wanted Suzanne to look at me before I looked and before I let Walker look at me. Suzanne was really nervous as Dr. Naman unwrapped the bandage. I watched her face the whole time. Then I saw the look of relief come over her face. "It's not bad! Really, I'm telling you the truth. It's not bad. Let me get a mirror," she said. I took the mirror and with trembling hands I held it up to see what I looked like. It wasn't bad at all. One breast was higher than the other but Dr. Naman said, "This left breast will settle down into position so they will be even." The stitches were all on the inside. No Frankenstein stitches, just thin neat lines. The nipples were gone, but like I said, I knew that was temporary. I was relieved. The nightmare was over. I thanked Dr. Naman for doing such a wonderful job.

"When can I go home?" I asked. "You can go home tomorrow if you feel like it," he said as he wrapped my chest up in a fresh bandage. That was a Thursday, just three days after my surgery. "My sister who lives in Savannah is having a family get together on Saturday. Do you think I could go? I'll just be sitting around talking to a bunch of relatives."

"I think you can. Just don't do anything strenuous. I have to leave to go to Mexico as soon as you're released. I'm doing some volunteer surgery down there. I hate to leave you, but if you have any trouble you can call Mac. Dr. Smith is about to leave town too," he said. I knew that both Dr. Naman and Dr. Smith were leaving town right after my surgery. I had asked them to go ahead and do my surgery before they left town because I didn't want that cancer to spread while they were gone. I was relieved that they went ahead and did my surgery before they left.

"Now let me show you how to deal with these drains. On each side you have two plastic tubes under your skin. They stick out of your skin and attached to each one is a plastic bulb to collect fluid that will be coming out of the wound. The bulbs have numbers printed on them so you can measure and record how much fluid is coming out of each drain before you open the bulb and discard the fluid. When it gets to the point that the drains have pretty much stopped putting out any fluid, I'll just pull the drains out. You think you can handle that?" Dr. Naman asked. "Oh, sure, no problem."

> **Girlfriend advice:** I had been told before the surgery that I could purchase a camisole that had pockets on each side to put the drain bulbs in. You can probably find one of these camisoles at the breast cancer boutique in the hospital where you are going to have your surgery. I bought mine at the breast cancer boutique at the John B. Amos Cancer Center. The sales ladies in the boutique were wonderful. They showed me how to place the drain bulbs in the camisole to make my post surgery life easier. Purchase your camisole before you have your surgery because you will need it as soon as you wake up from your surgery. That little camisole was great. It was well worth its weight in gold.

So I went home on Thursday and to tell you the truth draining those bulbs of their fluid was a royal pain in the neck. I don't know why, but the fluid just looked so disgusting, that when I tried to squeeze the fluid out of the bulbs, I would get very sick at my stomach. Luckily, good old Walker took over that job. I rested at home in Macon on Friday and on Saturday we took Laurel, Olivia, and Blythe with us to my sister Cea's house in Savannah. My surgery had only been six days before but I felt fine, no pain or discomfort. My chest was tightly bandaged, my drains were doing their thing, and I had a nice visit with my relatives. We stayed in a beautiful hotel in Savannah and had a great time. On Sunday we drove back home to Macon and all was well that night when I went to bed....

STAPH INFECTION. BACK INTO THE HOSPITAL.

Dear Girlfriend,

The next morning, Monday, I woke up having hard chills. I am talking about the worst chills I have ever had in my life. Even though it was June, I was freezing to death. I pulled the blankets up over me, and my body just drew up in a fetal position, while I shook so violently that the headboard on our old antique bed started rocking back and forth. My teeth were chattering. Walker was asleep beside me when the rocking headboard woke him up. He sat up in bed and asked, "What are you doing?" My teeth just kept on chattering like one of those toy sets of wind- up dentures and my body just scrunched up smaller and smaller.

Walker felt my forehead. I was burning up with fever. He jumped out of bed and ran to the bathroom, got the thermometer, and stuck it in my mouth. I had a hard time holding it in my mouth because my teeth kept on clacking. He took the thermometer out of my mouth and held it under the bedside lamp, "It's 105! You must have an infection. We have to get you to the hospital."

"I'm not going anywhere!" I said and hid under the covers. I was still shaking hard enough for the headboard to rock back and forth. "Oh, yes, you are!" he yelled as he ran around trying to get his clothes on and trying to find something for me to put on. "Just get me some Tylenol. I don't need to go to the hospital!" I managed to say through my chattering teeth. But before I knew what had happened, he had dressed me and was dragging me down the stairs. "Leave me alone. I'm fine. I don't need to go to the hospital!"

"Suzan, you are sick. Really sick. You have to go to the emergency room."

"I'll be alright in a little while. Please don't put me back in the hospital!"

He threw a blanket over me and led me out to the car. He called a dear family friend who is an emergency room doctor and told him we were coming. Our friend was not on duty, but he said he would make sure we were taken back immediately. We drove to the emergency room. The next thing I knew I was in some sort of holding room. By the time I got to the hospital my chills had stopped and my fever had gone down. I guess the Tylenol I took at home had kicked in. Compared to the other patients, I really didn't seem to be in an emergency situation.

After several hours of just watching me rest on an examination table, Walker found a nurse and explained to her that I had just had a bilateral mastectomy a few days before. Girlfriend, this is why you absolutely must have your advocate with you, not only when you go to your doctor's appointments, but also when you go to the hospital. This is especially true in an emergency room where there might be patients who appear to be in worse shape than you are, so of course the doctors will try to deal with them first. Walker suggested to the nurse that she take fluid out of the bulbs and culture it to see what was going on. The nurse had to go get an order from a doctor to do this. When she came back, she took fluid from one bulb attached to one of my drains on the right breast.

Walker, acting as my advocate said, "Take some fluid from her left breast too, that's the side that had cancer and radiation. If she has an infection it's probably coming from that left, weaker breast." If he had not been there, I would have never thought to give the nurse that information. In order to take fluid from my other breast, she had to go back and find a doctor to give her an order to drain fluid from the other breast. All this was taking a lot of time, giving the infection time to grow stronger and more difficult to get under control. Finally, the nurse did take fluid from both breasts and took it to the lab to be cultured.

While we were waiting for the lab report, the same nurse tried to take my blood pressure using my left arm. Again, Walker acting on my behalf said, "You need to take her blood pressure on the right arm, she's had fourteen lymph nodes removed from the left side." There again, I would not have thought to mention to the nurse that you can't take blood pressure from an arm on the same side where lymph nodes have been removed.

Then, after the lab report came back saying that I had an infection, the nurse tried to put an IV for an antibiotic into my port. Walker spoke up again and said, "That port was just installed a few days ago. The stitches haven't even healed yet. I don't think it's ready to be used." So, the nurse took blood to be tested from a vein in my arm, instead of using my port. Now girlfriend, just think, if I had not had Walker with me, there would have been nobody to guide that nurse with information she needed to take care of me. Nurses and doctors are only human, they can't read minds, and because I was so sick, I didn't feel like talking at all. Take your buddy with you to be your advocate when you are not up to talking to the caregivers yourself. The caregivers are happy to be told what is going on with you so they can better do their jobs. Sometimes they just don't have much information about you, unless you, or your advocate, speaks up and tells them what they need to know.

One of my dearest friends, Vera, a registered nurse,was on duty at the hospital. I had called her on my cell phone to tell her that I was down in the emergency room. After my blood was tested, she came in and held my hand. "Walker, she has a bad staph infection," she said. Before I knew what was going on they hooked me up to an IV with an antibiotic. The antibiotic they gave me was not very strong. They kept me in the emergency room all day long. Finally, about six o'clock in the afternoon, a doctor came in and told us that I was free to go, but to go see my primary care physician the next day. All through this story Walker was right by my side. He was my guardian.

Girlfriend advice: The breast cancer journey is hard. If you are not married, please enlist the help of a dear friend to go with you, not only to doctor's office appointments, but also to stay with you any time you are in the hospital. You need someone to look after you at all times!

When the emergency room doctor in Macon said that I could go home (but with no additional medication!!!), I was perfectly happy to go home, but Walker, acting with good judgment, which I did not have at that moment, called Dr. Mac Molnar in Columbus, since Dr. Smith and Dr. Naman were both out of town. Mac told Walker to put me in the car and drive me straight back to the hospital in Columbus as fast as he could get there. When we got to the hospital in Columbus, Mac was there to meet us.

He did more blood work and determined that I had a serious case of staph aureus. My white cell count was 19,000. Normal is around five to ten thousand. In other words, there was an extremely serious war going on inside my body. Think of your white cells as soldiers. When you do not have an infection, a normal number of soldiers are on patrol in your body. When your body is being attacked by an infection, such as staph, the troops are called in to fight the war. Mac could tell that I had a very serious staph infection because my white cell count, my soldier count, was extremely high. He decided to hit me with his best shot. He told the nurses to start me on an extremely strong antibiotic called Vancomycin.

I was so thankful that our dear friend, Mac, was there to take care of me. To tell you the truth, at that point, I really didn't think I was particularly sick. My chills had stopped and my fever had eased after I had taken the Tylenol. I had been in the emergency room in Macon all day long, so by the time we drove a hundred miles to Columbus and I got admitted to a room, it was about ten o'clock at night.

A nurse came in and said, "You were supposed to be in the bed by the window, but something is wrong with that bed, I can't get it to go down. It's stuck up so high and you are so little, I don't think you can get up on it easily. Just get in the other bed by the wall. Your husband can sleep in the high bed instead of that awful recliner. He'll be a lot more comfortable." We were so exhausted. I remember just plopping down on that bed while nurses hooked me up to an IV to administer the antibiotic. Poor Walker was so tired he just crawled into the broken bed by the window and was snoring away within a minute.

Even though I was so tired, after the nurses left I just lay there staring at the ceiling. I wasn't afraid because I really had no idea how seriously sick I was. About thirty minutes passed and I watched as two nice looking young nurses came in and approached Walker's bed. I thought that they were going to tell him he had to give up his comfy bed and go back to the recliner, but they were confused and thought that Walker was the patient. I just lay there and listened as one nurse woke him up and said in a sweet little voice, "Sir, I hate to bother you, but we need to check you from head to toe for pressure sores." Walker just turned over, got a big smile on his face and jokingly said, "Go right ahead!" I guess he thought two good looking women checking him out from head to toe was the most interesting activity he had seen in quite a while.

When I heard what he said, I popped up in my bed and said, "You old fool! You aren't even a patient!" At that the two nurses turned their attention to me and said, "Who are you?" I said, "I'm the patient. That's my husband and neither one of us has pressure sores because we've only been in bed about thirty minutes!" At that we all started laughing and they changed me to the bed by the wall on their chart.

When they left Walker said, "Well, it sounded like a good idea to me. I didn't mind them checking me out. You messed up their plan."

"Go to sleep!" I said as I curled up in my covers, " You're lucky they didn't mistake you for somebody who needed to have his leg cut off!"

"Now you've done it. I'll be awake all night long," he said as I drifted off to sleep....

A BATTLE GOING ON INSIDE OF ME.

Dear Girlfriend,

It was determined that the staph infection was in the left breast, the breast that had had cancer, the breast that had been severely weakened by twenty-eight radiation treatments. The days just rolled by and there was no significant change in my white blood cell count. I was one sick puppy. Mac called Dr. Naman in Mexico and told him what was going on. They discussed whether or not to just take out the implant until the infection was healed. I knew that if Mac took out the implant, then I would be without a breast on the left side . The thought of seeing myself with no breast was just more than I could stand. I told Mac that I wanted so badly to try to save the implant. He thought I should let him take it out, but I was so afraid of having no breast that he agreed to finish the round of the antibiotic and see what happened.

After I had taken all but the last two bags of Vancomycin, my white cell count was still 13,000. Mac came to my room that night and for the first time I could tell that he was really worried. Up until that point I really wasn't worried. I remember him sitting in a chair in my room looking at the internet on his cell phone. He had a furrowed brow and was thinking out loud as he looked at different treatments for staph. "Well, we could try this...or we could try that...." Then it really hit me. He was worried. The antibiotic was not working as well as he had hoped. We only had two bags left and I knew if that infection was not gone after those two bags were administered, he would insist on taking out the implant and I would have no breast on the left side.

"Well, let's just see how your blood work looks in the morning. Try to get some sleep," he said with a weary look on his face. Now, girlfriend, this is a part of my story that you may or may not choose to believe, but I promise you that I'm telling you the truth. When you have cancer, the big elephant that is always in the room, but is seldom mentioned is, "Am I going to die?" The second big elephant in the room is, "If I die, is there really life after death or will I just cease to exist? Will I stop having any awareness of anything, like before I was born? Will I just be gone forever, or will I go on to the next stage of life that is eternal?" These are scary questions.

I was raised in the Catholic faith. Some people think that Catholics have all kinds of peculiar beliefs. Actually, there are a few that I think are pretty peculiar myself. I guess anytime you have human beings organizing anything for two thousand years, you are bound to wind up with some rules or beliefs that are peculiar. It is in human nature to take something that is supposed to be very simple and turn it into something very complicated. Just look at our government for an example of that!

Most Catholics that I know don't believe every single thing that is in the four hundred pound Catechism of the Catholic Church. However, that is perfectly alright, because I had it said very clearly to me by an elderly Catholic priest, "Listen to your conscience. God will always tell you what is right. Love God with your whole heart, your whole mind and your whole soul. Love your neighbor as much as you love yourself. If you just concentrate on that, you won't have time to sweat the small stuff."

And you know, he was right. So I became a cafeteria Catholic. A cafeteria Catholic says, "Oh, I'll believe this, but I'm really not comfortable with that. Put some of that on my plate, but you can keep all of that!" And according to my old friend the priest, as long as you are sincerely following your conscience, the guiding voice of God inside of you, then you will do the right thing. God will never point you in the wrong direction no matter what all those man- made rules tell you to do.

God's one law, the only law, is to love God with your whole heart, your whole soul and your whole mind and love your neighbor as you love yourself. That one law, the only law, is pretty doggone hard to keep. Who do you know who loves every other person in the world as much as he loves himself? To tell you the truth, there are some people that I don't even like. I mean if one of those people fell in a deep hole, I would go find a rope to pull them out, but, after pulling them out, I just might not invite them back to my house for supper. And most people are probably like me. We just do the best we can, but we aren't perfect.

So after Mac left Walker and me alone in my hospital room that night, I lay there on the bed with that antibiotic dripping down into the vein in my hand and I thought about prayer. I thought about way way back in Catholic school when I was a child and we prayed to God. We prayed to saints and we prayed to angels and Sister Mary Amalia said, "Prayer is just talking to God. God is always there. You are never alone. He is always there." One child asked, "Sister, what is a saint?"

"Well, a saint is just someone who has left this life on earth, and gone to heaven to live with God."

"My grandmother died. Is she a saint?"

"If your grandmother loved God and was truly sorry for the sins she committed in her life, then when she died she went to heaven to live with God, so if that was the case, then yes, your grandmother is a saint. It's just very simple."

"Can I pray to my grandmother, Sister?"

"Of course you can. Praying is just talking to someone who has gone on to heaven. You can pray to your grandmother to ask her to pray for you. Saints are just people who have gone to heaven. St. Paul said that we are surrounded by a cloud of witnesses. That means that your loved ones who have passed away are all around you. I think that they can see you and look out for you. Heaven is not some far off place in the sky. It's all around you. All the people who have passed away are still right around you, you can talk to them, or pray to them, whatever you want to call it."

Remembering those childhood days I lay in the darkness with that IV dripping into me and I prayed. I prayed to God to make my white blood cell count go down to nine thousand. Nine thousand was the number Mac was looking for and I could not leave the hospital until my white cell count was at least down to nine thousand. Then I got an idea. Everyone I knew was praying for me... my brothers, my sisters, my friends, my husband, my children. What about asking people who were already in heaven to pray for me? What about asking Daddy to pray for me? What about asking my five girlfriends who had passed away from cancer to pray for me? What about asking the patron saint of breasts to pray for me?

In the Catholic church over the years there have been people who led such good lives, people who loved God so much and loved people so much that the Church just truly believed that these people went to heaven. In our day many people think that Mother Teresa, who worked with the poor sick people in India, must have gone to heaven when she passed away. And if she did, that would make her a saint. It is believed that some people who are in heaven have prayed with people who are still on Earth for particular kinds of help. These are called patron saints.

As I lay in the darkness attached to monitors and my IV of antibiotics, I remembered what that elderly priest told me. He said, "I think heaven must be like that movie *Ghost*. You know that movie with Whoopi Goldberg? I really like Whoopi Goldberg... Remember how the fellow that got murdered, Patrick Swayze...remember how he could see Demi Moore, but she couldn't see him? Patrick Swayze was trying to help Demi Moore because that bad guy was going to kill her too? Well, I think that is just how heaven is...it's like Patrick Swayze watching over Demi Moore and she didn't even know he was there. He was there, but she just couldn't see him. That's heaven! Our loved ones are watching over us, all around us, but we just can't see them... I just love that Whoopi Goldberg...."

I mulled all this over in my mind and then I sat up in bed, "Walker! Do you have your laptop with you? Can you get internet in here?"

"Yeah, I can get internet."

"Okay. Listen. I want you to look up the patron saint of breasts."

"The what?" Walker is a convert so some of this stuff is still news to him.

"The patron saint of breasts," I said.

"Are you serious? There's a patron saint of titties?"

"Breasts. There's a patron saint of everything. I want to ask her to join in with everybody else who's praying for me. I mean it might not help, but it sure couldn't hurt!" Walker got out of bed and got out his laptop. "I'm not believing this. You're right. There's a patron saint of breast cancer. St. Agatha. Wow. That's pretty cool," he said.

"Well, what does it say about her?" I asked.

"It says that she was martyred in Sicily in the year 251. She was a beautiful and wealthy Christian girl during the time of Roman persecution. A Roman judge, Quintian, asked her to marry him and renounce her Christian faith. He wanted her to worship the Roman gods. She refused, so he had her breasts cut off. Right before she died, she praised God, and asked to be with Him in eternity. She is the patron saint of women with breast cancer and women who have been sexually assaulted," he said.

"Wow. That makes what I'm going through sound better. I want to ask her to pray for me."

Walker came over and sat on the edge of my bed. He took my hand that had the IV in it. I just remember saying, "Dear Saint Agatha, please pray for me. Please ask God to make my white cell count go down to nine thousand. Dear Lord, please hear my prayer and the prayers of all the other people who are praying for me to be cured from this infection that is trying to kill me. Amen."

"There's a prayer on the internet that's really nice. Let me read it to you. 'Oh, heavenly Father, Who raised Agatha to the dignity of sainthood, we implore your Divine Majesty, by her intersession to give us health of mind, body and soul. Free us from all those things which hold us to this earth and let our spirits like hers, rise to your heavenly courts. Through Jesus Christ our Lord who lives and reigns with you forever. Amen.'" Walker closed his laptop and kissed me on the top of my head. Then he climbed back into the high bed and we both went to sleep.

The next morning a nurse came and drew my blood. In a while we received word from Mac that my white cell count was exactly where it needed to be, nine thousand, normal. "I think God answered our prayers," I told Walker as he squeezed my hand. Then a lady from the office came in and told us that since my white cell count was normal, my insurance provider wanted me to leave the hospital immediately. "But she still has one more bag to be administered in the morning. We can't stop the antibiotic before the end of the regimen or the infection might just come right back! This is crazy!" Walker got Mac on the phone and he went to the office to talk to the lady in charge of insurance. She decided that since the last bag of antibiotic had to be administered promptly at 5:30 A.M., and since there were no outpatient facilities that could provide the service on that schedule, I could stay to finish the treatment. So the next morning at 5:30 A.M. I received the final bag of Vancomycin and then a nurse came with a wheel chair to roll me right out the door just as soon as the bag was empty. I had been in the hospital nine days. As Walker and the nurse helped me get into the car, I thought about that prayer he had read on the internet, "Lord, give us health of mind, body and soul...free us from those things that hold us to this earth...."

THE LIGHT, WHICH IS GOD, WAS SHINING OUT OF HIM.

Dear Girlfriend,

After we left the hospital, we drove directly to the office of my plastic surgeon, Dr. Naman. He had just returned from Mexico. As he examined me he said, "When I talked to Mac while I was in Mexico I was so worried about you. Your incision, however, still looks good. Maybe you'll be able to keep the implant in now that the infection is gone." I was so happy to hear him say that.

After we left Dr. Naman's office we went directly to see my oncologist Dr. Pippas. He came in and shook my hand. He shook Walker's hand. He was not even smiling. He sat down and started to read my pathology report. Dr. Naman had told me while I was still in the hospital that there was no more cancer found in my left breast when it was removed. Dr. Pippas was reading the report for the first time and finally I saw him get excited and grin from ear to ear, "This is miraculous! This is miraculous! Dr. Smith got it all when he did the biopsy. There was no more cancer found in the breast tissue that was removed! This is miraculous!" I was so excited that he was so excited. Up until that point I was really intimidated by him because he was so so serious. I know cancer is serious, but a smile is the light, which is God, shining out of you. I was so happy to finally see that light shining out of Dr. Pippas.

We went home and I decided to keep on resting in the bed. I had this nightgown that actually looked like something that would have been issued to an inmate in prison. It was striped, it was ugly, but it was so soft that I just kept on washing it and wearing it.

Word had gotten out about how sick I had been and the casserole brigade started up once more. "This is great!" Walker said as he wolfed down a broccoli chicken casserole. "How long is this gonna go on? Janet said she's bringing dinner and a pound cake and Carole is bringing a chocolate cake. Becky and Kitty are bringing the dinner on Wednesday and Leslie on Thursday. Julie is bringing chicken tetrazzini and Suzanne is bringing shrimp pasta on Friday. Molly brought yogurt and fruit and Vera brought flowers. Look at all this food! You need to stay in bed at least a month!" It was overwhelming. I couldn't believe how many people had sent cards, food, flowers and prayers my way.

I just lay up in the bed like Miss Astor while friend after friend came to my bedside to keep me company. Then the e-mail came. Walker just casually mentioned that this cute little divorcee had sent him an e-mail asking about my health. "Why did she e-mail you? She has my e-mail address," I asked. "Oh, I don't know, she probably didn't want to bother you." I looked in the mirror on my bedside table at my ugly nightgown. No makeup. Hair needed coloring. "Well, I'm not dead yet!" I told Walker as I pushed myself out of the bed and went to look for something decent to put on. "You're jealous!" he said.

"Well, I love all my girlfriends bringing me goodies, but she's just a buzzard circling around waiting for me to croak!" I said.

"You're being ridiculous."

"And you're being naive! Walker, you'd be a good catch. You're rugged and good looking, and you live in a mansion.... I'm getting out of bed!"

"You're so funny. That girl was just concerned about you."

"Well, I'm concerned about me too. She's too good looking for me to be looking like this!" I was scooting around the room grabbing up clothes and makeup, a hair brush and a hair dryer. " I'll see you later!" I said as I backed into the bathroom.

I took off my nightgown and looked at myself in the mirror. Ugh. The implant that was on the left side, the side that had cancer, was just not healing. It was quite a bit higher than the other breast and it felt very hard. The incision looked fresh, like I had just had surgery, even though it had been about three weeks. Surprisingly, not having nipples did not look bad. I had thought that would be disgusting, but it wasn't bad. I just kept telling myself that new and maybe prettier ones were coming soon. Unfortunately, it was becoming evident that I had so much radiation damage that my skin was thin and weak. Add a serious staph infection on top of the radiation damage, and I had a very bad situation.

The incision looked stressed, as if it could rip out at any minute. I washed my hair leaning over the bathtub. I dried my hair and put on makeup and a soft cotton knit dress. I felt better, but when I looked at myself in the mirror, I knew that something very basic about me had changed. Something very basic about my personality had changed. Let me see if I can put this into words. Before I had my breasts removed, I was not afraid. I was not afraid of life. I never thought about death. After I had my breasts removed it was like I had joined a secret society. This secret society was made up of the people who had experienced personal tragedy that was so great that they were never quite the same again.

Having cancer took away my innocence. It took away my carefree mind. It made me feel shaken, like if this could happen, anything bad could happen. A strange feeling of mourning came over me. One day I happened to be looking through some papers on Walker's desk, I came across the pathology report from my surgery. It said that my breasts were in two jars labeled left and right. It said that my nipples were in two jars labeled left and right. Then I realized why I had felt so much grief after my breasts were removed. I was actually mourning for my breasts.

The reason I am sharing this with you is to let you know that this is perfectly normal. But, even more importantly, I want to let you know that in time the pain does get better. The fear of "What horrible thing is going to happen next?" will get better. And most important of all, with this deep mourning will come a new and clearer understanding of other people's pain. Since I had experienced such a great loss, I became more able to understand the walking wounded in my life.

The first person that I came to understand better was my own mother. My mother is now ninety-one years old. Mary Josephine Pacetty was born in 1921. She was an exceptionally beautiful girl. She grew up in Columbus, Georgia, the youngest of her parents' four daughters. Her father and mother doted on her. Her father was a portrait photographer, and after school when she was a little girl, she would walk to his studio. She would play dress up in the costumes that were there for the people who were having their picture taken. Her daddy loved her so much that he took tons of pictures of his darling little girl. She would hang around waiting for her daddy to close the studio and then they would walk home together. Her dog, Easy, would wait on the corner for them and when he saw her approaching he would run with his wagging tail to greet her.

When she was just a girl of twenty, spending her time going to dances with her many young suitors and enjoying the best time of her life, a terrible tragedy happened. Her daddy, whom she was so close to, along with both of her older married sisters' little girls, were killed in a car wreck by a drunk driver. My mother, a carefree beautiful young spirit just twenty years old, had to experience seeing the bodies of her three-year-old niece, her seven-year- old niece, and her beloved daddy laid out in the family parlor. From all that she has shared with me, this tragedy changed her to her very core.

She was afraid for the rest of her life. She was always thinking ahead about what bad thing could happen next. She became reclusive and a chronic worrier. She was not the carefree girl that she had been before. The reason I am telling you this is so you will be careful.

Girlfriend advice: Yes, having cancer might shake you to your very core. You might not ever feel as safe in the world as you did before, but don't let that ruin your life. Don't let yourself be reclusive. Even if you really don't want to be around people, go out anyway.

When you feel your mind drifting into a dark place where there is fear of death, pray. Pray that you will have the strength to control your fear. Pray to the Holy Spirit to dwell in you. Pray that the Holy Spirit will bring you peace of mind and a healthy body. Write a journal and don't be afraid to express your deepest darkest fears. Writing will get that pain out of you. You can confide in your friends who have also had breast cancer and they, like nobody else, will know how you are feeling and they will help you get through it.

I have a dear friend named Laura who has had the exact same path through her breast cancer journey as I had. She is just a few steps ahead of me in her treatment, so, whenever she has a procedure, we get together for a five hour lunch and talk it all out. She tells me what I can expect to happen next. Seeing that her hair did grow back, and her lovely figure did come back after reconstruction, has been a God send to me. If you don't have a girlfriend that has had a similar breast cancer experience, then ask your doctor to call one of his patients and ask her if he can give you her name. Believe me, one of the "sisters" will be happy to be your new friend.

By having cancer you have joined the ranks of the walking wounded. I think that there are very few, if any people, who don't eventually join the ranks of the walking wounded. When I had my breasts removed, I was taken in by one friend who had recently lost a child. I was just blown away that she was coming and taking me to lunch on a regular basis after what she had been through. I was taken in by another friend who had been sexually molested. I was taken in by many people who had had their own personal tragedies, and somehow, having gone through so much pain themselves, had made them kinder and gentler and more understanding of my pain and they surrounded me with their love. Now I feel as if it is my turn to pass on the peace they gave me to you.

That is what this book is about, my trying to pass peace to you. I cannot honestly say that I have completely conquered my fear of death, but I can say it is better. What I can say is keep holding on to the fact that every stage of this painful journey is only temporary and if you will let them in, many women will be there to help you on your way. So as I came out of my prison nightgown and back into regular clothes and makeup, I knew that outwardly I looked about the same to other people, but inwardly I was a different person. Yes, I had been shaken to the core. Yes, I had joined the ranks of the walking wounded, but I had also calmed down. I was more able to see other people as wounded and not judge them as harshly as I had before. Even people that I didn't like, even people who had hurt me deeply, I started to feel less hard toward. I let go of a lot of my unforgiving feelings because I started to see that they were wounded too....

And for that reason, being wounded by cancer helped me to become a better person. This time on Earth is all about reaching our highest potential. For me, cancer pushed me way down the road and I became a kinder, more understanding, less judgmental person. And that is one good thing that came out of my having cancer. You also have to make a decision, girlfriend, you can decide to take the nightmare that is cancer and learn from it and grow into a better person, or you can let cancer destroy you, not only physically, but also mentally and spiritually You have freewill. You make the decision.

LOVED ONES IN HEAVEN ARE WATCHING OVER ME.

Dear Girlfriend,

During the month of July, 2010, Walker, my three daughters and I went to St. Augustine, Florida, for a much needed vacation. When I said earlier that the big elephant in the room is, "Will I die and just cease to exist?" I really meant what I said. Everybody who has ever lived has asked themselves that question. No matter how strong your faith is, I feel that most people who have a life threatening disease, are still afraid of the unknown, death. I want to share an experience with you that I had. This incredible experience made me believe that we do not cease to exist after we pass away. This experience put me more at ease with the thought of the eventual inevitability of the the the end of this stage of life.

I have always been interested in tracing my family tree. My mother's maiden name is Pacetty. Her father's family first came to Florida from Sicily and Minorca in the late 1700's to work as indentured servants on an indigo plantation, located about ninety miles from what is now St. Augustine, Florida. I had always heard growing up that the Pacetty's had come from St. Augustine, but I really didn't know much about their story. About ten years ago, Walker and I made a trip to St. Augustine to do a little research on my family history.

We were staying out on the beach in a rented condo. I didn't know one living soul in St. Augustine, so I just picked up the phone book and looked up the name Pacetti. I knew that was the old spelling of Pacetty. My ancestor had changed the spelling of his name from Pacetti to Pacetty for reasons I will never know. When I looked up Pacetti in the St. Augustine phone book, there were sixty-four listings. I didn't know where to start so I just randomly picked one. As it turned out, the gentleman who answered the phone, just happened to be the mayor of St. Augustine Beach. I told him who I was and what I was doing and he was just as nice as he could be. He ran a real estate company and he told me to come on over and meet him. So Walker and the girls and I went to meet my very distant relative, Mr. Pacetti.

I was so happy and excited to meet this relative of mine and he was just as happy and excited to meet us. I asked him if he knew any stories about the Pacetti family history. He said, "I'm really not the one you need to talk to. You need to talk to my great aunt. She's keeps up with all the Pacetti stories. She lives in the old home place out on Pacetti Road."

I was so impressed that there was actually a Pacetti Road. So he called her on the phone and she said that she would love for us to come meet her. What an adventure! We said our fond farewells to our newly found relative, piled in the car and set out to find Pacetti Road. Sure enough we found Aunt Pacetti living out in the country in an old frame house. She welcomed us warmly and we told her we were looking for information about the Pacetti family.

She told us many interesting stories and I was just thrilled to hear every word she said. Then she told us what I thought was the most interesting story of all. "Back in the 1830's, the Pacetti family lived in a log cabin on this very same land. The Pacetti women became friends with the Indian women in the area. When the Indian babies got sick, their mothers would bring them to the Pacetti women because they knew the Pacetti women would help them. Then in 1838 the U.S. Government tried to take the land away from the Seminoles. They wanted the Indians to move to some territory west of the Mississippi River."

"Was that the conflict that Osceola got involved in?" I asked.

"Yes, it was. You see Osceola encouraged the Indians to fight back. So some Indian women went to the Pacetti's cabin and warned them. They told the Pacetti's to leave their cabin because the Indians were going to burn down all the white people's cabins. So your ancestor, Andrew Pacetti, took his family and went into the town of St. Augustine and they hid out in Fort Marion (now commonly known as Castillo de San Marcos). Osceola was captured, and after things had calmed down, Andrew Pacetti took his family and went home. All along the way they saw their neighbors' cabins and crops that had been burned. They just knew their cabin was going to be burned down too. But, when they got there, they discovered that the cabin had not been touched. Evidently, the Indian women told the Indian men to leave the Pacetti home place alone, because the Pacetti's had been so good to them."

That story just gave me goosebumps. Now, fast forward to July, 2010. Walker and I took the girls to go tour the old fort in St. Augustine, where the Pacetti's supposedly hid out according to Aunt Pacetti. If you have never been to Fort Marion, in St. Augustine, let me tell you it is just one huge storage room after another. These rooms are tremendous and have no windows, so they are extremely dark. The only light that enters the room is through the door. We wandered from storage room to storage room and through some rooms that had been used as barracks. Then we entered a huge room that was next to what had been the chapel. As soon as we entered that room, I remembered what Aunt Pacetti had told us about my ancestor, Andrew Pacetti, taking his family to hide out in the fort during the Indian uprising.

I got the strangest feeling as I walked into what had been the chapel. I saw the ancient altar and a niche carved out of the wall where a statue must have been. And then I imagined people, scared people huddled together, praying for safety. They were praying that their homes and their lives would be spared. And then I just knew. I knew that if the story Aunt Pacetti told me was true, this was where my ancestors would have hidden in this fort. They would not have hidden in the barracks. They would not have hidden in a room where ammunition was stored. They would have hidden in or near the chapel. I walked out of the chapel back into the large holding room beside it. If the story was true, I knew this was where they would have slept. They would have been all huddled together, sleeping on the hard floor. I could just see in my mind how it would have been. Andrew Pacetti, his wife, Catherine, and their little children huddled up on the floor with their friends and neighbors and strangers too, all scared to death.

The room I stood in was dark. The only light came through the small door. The ceiling was at least twenty feet high. The walls were scratched up with hundreds of years of abuse. I stood there in that room and in my mind I said, "Andrew Pacetti, if you were here, if the story was true, let me know! Let me know that God has kept you alive in heaven! Please Andrew, help me overcome my fear of death!" At that very moment I felt as if someone took me by the shoulders and turned me around, and there, with the light from the doorway shining on the wall was scratched in letters six inches tall, "A. Pacetti."

I felt a thrill I can't even describe. I grabbed Walker by the arm and told him what had happened as I pointed to the name on the wall. He took his camera and started taking pictures of it and then I realized a group of tourists were listening to what I had said. They were all smiling and taking pictures of it too. Yes, cancer is powerfully destructive, but fear not, it can not destroy the power of the resurrection. It cannot destroy the power of eternal life....

YOU MEAN I'M DEAD???

Dear Girlfriend,

When we got back to Macon from our trip to Florida, my oncologist, Dr. Pippas, ordered a test called a Muga Scan. I was told that I needed to start chemo just as soon as my incisions were healed because chemo is the most effective if it is done within six months after the surgery. My problem was that my left breast, the side on which I had had cancer , was just not healing. After six weeks that left breast still looked just like it had right after surgery. But, I went ahead to the hospital to have the Muga Scan, a test to determine if one's blood is pumping throughout the body properly. It's important that your blood is pumping normally if you are going to do chemotherapy. The Muga Scan does not hurt. It's done at a nuclear medicine center or by a radiology tech at the hospital. You don't eat or drink anything for four to six hours before the scan and you don't use caffeine or tobacco for four to six hours before the scan. Also, remember to wear comfy clothes because you are going to be lying on a table for a couple of hours.

Before the test, the technician will inject a little bit of radioactive material into a vein in your arm. This material is sort of like dye and it will hook up with your red blood cells as they carry oxygen through your body. See, like I told you, you are on automatic. When you woke up this morning, did you say, "Okay, red blood cells, get to work and take the oxygen I'm breathing all through my body. Chop! Chop! Get to it!" No. You didn't give your red blood cells one little thought because God is controlling all the inner workings of your body, just as surely as he holds the stars in the sky and keeps you from floating off the planet by controlling the force of gravity. But, do we ever think about any of that? Heck no!

So the technician had me lie on a table and she said, "This thing up above you is a gamma camera that uses gamma rays to take pictures of how blood is going through your heart. This won't hurt, but try to lie as still as you can or the pictures will be blurry and we'll have to do it over. I'll leave you here for a few minutes. Just relax, nothing will hurt you."

So I just lay there and thought about my blood traveling through my veins. I thought about the camera taking pictures of my heart. I was warm and cozy and unafraid until... the technician came back into the room and with no trace of a smile on her face she said, "I'm so sorry. You flatlined."

I jumped up off the table and shrieked, "You mean I'm dead???!!!" She started laughing and said, "Well, obviously not!" I could hardly breathe and I said, "But you said I flatlined, doesn't that mean I died?" She said, "I'm so sorry! I mean the machine stopped working. The machine flatlined." I lay back down on the table and said, "You scared me to death. I thought I had died, but just hadn't zooped up yet!" She said, "Well, I'll try to choose my words more carefully next time." We both had a good laugh, but I 'll bet she never told anybody else that they had "flatlined." My test came back normal, but I could not start chemo because my incisions had still not healed.

NO COINCIDENCE

Dear Girlfriend,

One morning soon after my Muga Scan, as I drank my coffee and read the newspaper, I came across an article about melanoma. This article said that the rule has always been, that if you have a mole that is as big as a pencil eraser, has irregular edges and color that is varied, you need to have it removed. This article said that now researchers say don't wait until the mole is as big as a pencil eraser. Even if your mole is teeny tiny, but has irregular edges and varied color, get it removed. I put my coffee cup down and went into my bedroom. I got my magnifying glass and looked at a teeny tiny little mole that was on my breast skin. It was not even as big as one half of a pencil eraser, but it was irregular in shape and had varied coloration that I could see with my magnifying glass. Now, I'm here to tell you again, listen to your inner feelings. I just stared at that tiny little mole that I couldn't even see clearly without a magnifying glass and there came another overwhelming feeling. That feeling was saying, "Get that mole removed!"

So I called Cheryl at Dr. Naman's office and made an appointment to have this miniscule mole removed. Dr. Naman removed the mole and sent it off to be tested. Guess what. It was the kind of mole that turns to melanoma. Melanoma is a deadly cancer if it goes internally, so Dr. Naman had me return to his office and he took more tissue just to make sure he had gotten rid of any precancerous cells. Now, what if I had not seen that article in the paper? What if I had not had that mole removed? I could be dead right now from melanoma. Somebody was definitely watching over me.... When something happens that gives you protection, don't think of it as coincidence. I very rarely get my news from the newspaper. Why was I reading that paper that morning? Why did that article attract my attention? There are no coincidences. There are just the loving arms of God around you.... Get the clutter out of your mind. Sit quietly. Listen to the voice of God deep inside you. He will hold your hand and guide you through cancer, if you will just listen to your feelings and let those feeling guide your decisions.

RADIATION DAMAGE. IMPLANT REMOVED.

Dear Girlfriend,

A few days later I was looking at my left breast with a mirror when I noticed that the skin had pulled apart and I could see something black. Quickly I called and made an appointment with Dr. Naman. He looked at my breast and said, "What we're seeing is the implant. I'm going to have to stitch it back up. So on August 3, 2010, I had yet another surgery, number six, to stitch up my implant. I went home and was super careful not to do anything that might cause it to rip again. Three weeks passed and I drove my car to the mall for the first time since June. As I was driving home, I looked down and noticed there was blood on my shirt. I called Dr. Naman and on August 24, 2010, I was back in the surgery center having another operation, number seven, to again stitch the implant back into my breast.

I was so careful, but no matter what I did or didn't do, that radiated skin was just not healing. I went to a dermatologist in Macon to see if he had any ideas on how to make the skin heal, but nothing he tried worked. Then the dermatologist suggested that I go to a hyperbaric wound healing center. So I talked to Dr. Naman about it and he made an appointment for me.

On the day of my appointment at the center, the doctor came in and examined my breast that absolutely refused to heal. "I think you could benefit from hyperbaric oxygen therapy, I want you to go on a tour of our facility and then set up a schedule of treatments with us."

He handed me over to a friendly nurse who took Walker and me into a room that made me feel as if I were in some sort of spaceship movie. Around the room there were people lying in clear plastic tubes about seven feet long. The room was dimly lit and the people were looking at a television that was mounted on the wall. The nurse explained to us, "The chambers were gradually pressurized with pure oxygen. We tell the patients to just relax and breathe normally. They're not in any discomfort. We have raised the pressure in the chamber to 2.5 times the normal atmospheric pressure. Most patients stay in the chamber from about thirty minutes to two hours a day. Each prescribed treatment is different. The chambers have to be depressurized before they are opened. What kind of wound do you have?"

"I'm having trouble with my skin healing after radiation for breast cancer," I said.

The nurse looked at me with concern, "If I were you... I wouldn't do this treatment... unless you are absolutely sure that there is no more cancer left in your body."

"But the doctor just said he thought I would be a good candidate for the treatment, and you know there really isn't any way we can be positive that all the cancer is gone," I replied.

"Well, I'm just telling you what I think." She showed us out to the lobby and the receptionist asked me if I wanted to set up a schedule for treatments. "I think I want to think about this for a while first," I said as I walked out the door. "Walker, what do you think? I mean that was a little weird. The doctor said he thought it would probably be good for me and the nurse said for me not to do it."

"I haven't got a clue. I'm totally confused," he said.

I went home and got on the internet. According to the American Cancer Society website , "The Food and Drug Administration (FDA) has approved HBOT to treat more than a dozen health problems such as decompression sickness, carbon monoxide poisoning, gangrene, brain abscess, and injuries in which tissues are not getting enough oxygen". I found some evidence that hyperbaric oxygen therapy was beneficial to soft tissue that had been damaged by radiation, but I just could not get what that nurse told me out of my head. So I just tried to relax and listen to my inner feelings, and to tell you the truth, I just felt too uncomfortable about doing the oxygen treatments. Now, girlfriend, I am not a doctor, or a nurse, so I'm not going to recommend or discourage you from using hyperbaric oxygen therapy. Discuss it with your doctor if you are having trouble with radiated skin that will not heal. As far as I'm concerned, I have no idea if it is good for cancer patients or not. I backed off from doing it because the nurse made me feel like it might cause my cancer to come back.

I went back home and continued to try to not do anything that would cause my skin to rip open again. After a couple of weeks, I opened the sliding door on the back of my house. The front of my shirt was immediately covered in blood. Dr. Naman stitched me up again, surgery number eight, but I was starting to feel like there was just no way that radiated skin was going to heal. On September 20, 2010, since there was still no sign of the breast healing, I went to Dr. Naman's surgery center for the implant to be removed. This was my ninth surgery.

He had tried so very hard to save the implant because he knew that I was terrified of being without my left breast. I was so afraid of looking hideous. When the surgery was over, Walker and I went up to our little cottage on Pine Mountain. Fairy Ring Cottage, nestled so far back in the forest, had been a place of refuge and healing for me. I was not nauseated or in any physical pain, so I just crawled under the covers and went to sleep. I slept all day long.

When I woke up, I was very depressed. After nine surgeries, twenty-eight radiation treatments and battling a deadly staph infection, I still had lost my breast implant. I knew I could not start chemotherapy until my skin was all healed and I couldn't do the latissimus flap surgery, where the tissue would be taken out of my back to build a breast, until my skin healed. I stayed at the cottage for a few days waiting for my surgery followup appointment with Dr. Naman. The night before I had my appointment with Dr. Naman to have my bandages taken off we were still at Fairy Ring Cottage.

I wanted to look at myself, without my breast, before I went to Dr. Naman's office, so I went in the bathroom and locked the door. I thought, "I can do this. It won't be that bad. How bad can it be? I'll just be without a breast for a few months while I do chemo. Then I can have the reconstruction taking the tissue out of my back. That won't be so bad. Slowly I took off my nightgown and just stood at the bathroom sink with nothing on but my panties. My chest was wrapped up in an Ace bandage.

When I looked at myself in the mirror over the sink, I remember thinking that I looked so white. My face looked like it had just fallen. I thought, "Okay. Just take a peek. The bandage is coming off tomorrow, so just take a little peek." My breast was covered with a thick white pad, like a sanitary napkin, that had been taped down with very wide tape. That pad gave the illusion that there was still something there. I thought in my naïve little mind that somehow, something, must still be there because the padding made it look full.

I started to pull the tape and the padding back, so I could take just a little peek. Then I saw it. For most women who have had a mastectomy, the skin is smooth and there is just a straight incision. But because I had had a very large implant in for three months, my skin was all stretched and "tacked up." In the middle of this tangled mess, there was a plastic drain to drain off any discharge from the wound. This plastic drain that looked like a small hose, was sticking out of a hole in my chest about the size of a nickel. Out of this hole in my chest was oozing a light green discharge. It was absolutely hideous.

Girlfriend, the reason I am telling you the truth and not sugar coating this description is because I want to be honest to prepare you for what you might see. Look at some pictures of women who have had to have an implant removed if you need to have your implant removed. I wish I had looked at some photographs of how I would look after the implant was removed, so that I could have been a little more prepared for what I saw. I had not seen any photographs and I was totally unprepared for what I looked like. I just stood there at the sink and screamed. I just remember holding on to the edge of the sink and hearing the sound of my own cry, as if I were some wounded animal caught in a steel trap. I knelt down on the cold tile floor and just held on to the sink and sobbed and sobbed.

I could hear Walker banging on the bathroom door, "Suzan! What happened?! Are you okay? Open the door! Open the door!" I didn't want to open the door. I wanted the floor to just swallow me up. I wanted to just disappear from this hellish nightmare that had become my life. I was sick to death of everything that just went on and on and on... Surgery after surgery. Fear. Needles. Infection. Vomit. Tears. I just wanted the floor to swallow me up. "Boo Boo! Open the door!" he sounded frantic. I pulled myself up on the sink and opened the door. Walker grabbed me and held me tight as I cried and blubbered, "I'm hideous!I'm disgusting! Don't look at me!!!!!!!"

Walker pulled me out of the bathroom and dragged me over to the bed. I lay down and once again I curled up in a little ball and cried. He once again curled up behind me and once again put his arms around me as I once again cried myself to sleep.....The next morning when I woke up, I knew I had to go to Dr. Naman's office to have the bandage completely taken off. I don't even remember the drive from Fairy Ring Cottage down to Columbus. When we got to Dr. Naman's office, Debbie called me to go back to the examination room. I usually talked and joked around with Debbie and Cheryl, the receptionist. All the girls in Dr. Naman's office have been so kind to me, but that morning I was not in a joking mood.

While Debbie stood holding the door open for me, I turned to Walker and said, "I don't want you to go back with me. I don't want you to see how awful I look." I got up and followed Debbie back to my same room. "Debbie, I peeked at myself. I look awful," I said. She said, "I know." I could have kissed her. If she had said, "It's not so bad !" I would have been hurt. I would have been angry. She said just exactly what I needed to hear. I didn't want to hear anybody lie to me and say, "Oh, it's not so bad...." She knew it was bad and I appreciated that she didn't trivialize what I was going through by saying, " Oh it's not so bad...."

Dr. Naman came in with a young female doctor from Russia. He was very kind as he took off the bandage completely. I asked for a mirror and got my first good look at myself. The tears came all over again. I just sobbed. I didn't know the doctor from Russia from Adam, but she was a woman and my instincts turned me to her. "I look hideous! How am I supposed to have sex looking like this? I'm disgusting! I'm gross!" She took my hand. It didn't matter that she was from the other side of the world, she was a woman and she felt sympathy for me.

I turned to Dr. Naman and said through my running nose and running mascara, "I have never seen anything on a human being that looks worse!" He just said, "I have." Then I thought about all the awful things he must have seen while doing his volunteer work in Mexico. Cleft palates. Amputated limbs. I felt ashamed of myself for saying what I had said. I immediately grabbed onto my life line, "This is only temporary! This is only temporary!" I thought of all the people in the world who are permanently disfigured in places on their bodies that there is no way to hide. I knew that I could hide my chest and my disfigurement would only be temporary. I also knew that I should feel very blessed.

Dr. Naman said, "I know this is hard on you because you're pretty, when you're not crying. You have a nice figure and you wear beautiful clothes. You really care about the way you look." He was so compassionate to have realized that I did care very much about the way I looked, but I didn't feel pretty anymore. That feeling had been gone for many years, and right now I just felt like I was repulsive and yes, that was very hard for me.

"Where is Walker?" he asked. "He's in the waiting room. I don't want him in here. I don't want him to look at me. I don't want him to be disappointed," I said.

"But he loves you. He comes to every appointment. That's really unusual. He won't be disappointed. Let's let him in."

"I love him too, so I don't want him to see how ugly I look."

"Let's let him in."

The Russian doctor handed me a Kleenex. I wiped my nose and said, "You can let him in, but I don't want him to look at me." Dr. Naman told the nurse to go get Walker. He came in and sat in his same chair. I covered myself up with the cloth bib and said, "Don't look at me!" Dr. Naman said, "She's afraid you'll be disappointed." Walker just looked kind of shell shocked and said, "I won't be disappointed."

I had to take the bib off so Dr. Naman could show me how to care for my wound. Walker turned his chair around and faced the wall. He didn't look. Not once.

Girlfriend advice: Go ahead and look at some pictures of what you will look like without a breast implant. Like I said, most women will just have a smooth, thin incision. My case was extraordinarily bad looking. Prepare yourself for what you will see when your bandage is removed. Let this be your mantra, "This is only temporary. This is only temporary. This is only temporary." Some women, who are okay with having just a smooth thin incision, opt to not have reconstruction. If you feel comfortable without reconstruction then bravo for you! Feeling comfortable is the name of the game!

I wanted reconstruction because I knew that I would feel better about myself with reconstruction. Now, since you have read that horrible part of the story, I feel as if I must tell you now, reconstruction can bring you back to look really good. It is awful getting there, but I know you can do it! Don't give up! The Pretty Titty Fairy will come visit you if that is what you want. Just hang in there and don't give up. Things are going to get better. The choice is yours! Insurance will pay for your reconstruction if you choose that path.

A BREAST MADE OUT OF GRITS???

Dear Girlfriend,

After I left Dr. Naman's office, I realized very quickly that I needed something to hide the fact that I was totally flat on my left side, so Walker and I went to the breast cancer boutique at the John B. Amos Cancer Center. The sweet young lady who waited on me was terrific. She told me that my insurance would pay for a breast prosthesis and four bras, but that she would have to order them and it would take at least a week for my order to come in. She measured me for the prosthesis and showed me the selection of bras. They were really pretty. I was pleasantly surprised. The bras looked just like any other bra except there was a pocket inside the bra for me to slip in the prosthesis. I was happy to hear that because I could just imagine that thing jumping out of the top of my bra and landing on the floor at a cocktail party. Then what would you say? Ta Dah!!! But, it seems that they think of everything. The friendly saleslady showed me bathing suits that had the same pocket so my prosthesis could not escape in the pool. What a relief!

I ordered the prosthesis and bras and was able to take a bathing suit home with me. When I got home I realized that I could wear a sports bra for the sake of comfort, but what could I stuff into the left side so I wouldn't look flat? I looked through my dresser drawers and found a sock. A friend of mine suggested that I fill the sock with couscous. Being a southern girl I decided to fill up the sock with dry grits. This actually could have worked pretty well except that I had that big hole in my chest that had not healed, so the grits felt too heavy against me.

Then eureka! I got a great idea. "Walker, will you go to the store and buy me a box of sanitary napkins? I'm going to try to use them for a breast." Walker just shook his head as he walked out the door to go to the grocery store to buy said sanitary napkins. Now girlfriend, before my breasts were removed, I wore a "D" cup, and so Dr. Naman had put my implants back the same size. My right breast, the one that was never radiated was healing nicely. So of course I wanted to use a large sanitary napkin on the left side so that they would match.

Then in comes Walker from the store with a package of mini pads that were about one eighth of an inch thick. I said, "Walker! What were you thinking? This pad is about as flat as a piece of paper!"

"Well, I don't know anything about those things! There were about fifty different kinds so I just grabbed one."

"Well, I will have to use at least six of these flat things to do the trick." So that's what I did. I just unwrapped about six or eight pads and stuck one on top of the next until both sides looked even. Necessity breeds invention. I swear, you never know where a day is going to take you....

Girlfriend advice: Talk to your doctor and see if there is any way that you can order your breast prosthesis before you have surgery. If you have your prosthesis when you leave the hospital, you will not have to create a temporary prosthesis.

SHE WHUPPED A HEALING ON HER!

Dear Girlfriend.

As I've said before, my mother lives in an assisted living home. I usually drive to Columbus twice a week to see her. Well, before I went into the hospital, I told the director of the home and a couple of Mama's favorite caregivers that I had cancer and was about to undergo surgery. I remember telling this one particular caregiver, I'll call Sally, that I was going into the hospital and I might not be able to see Mama for a few days. She hugged me and said that she would pray for me.

Now I have a sister, Cea, who is twelve years older than I am. We look very much alike except that Cea is older. So I had my surgery and staph infection and immediately went back to visit Mama, but I just didn't run into Sally for two or three weeks. She must have been working on the night shift. So in the meanwhile my sister, Cea, came from Virginia to visit Mama. When Sally ran into Cea in the hall of the home she thought Cea was me. She got a horrified look on her face as much to say, "I can sure tell you've been sick! You've aged ten years in the past few weeks!" Then she took Cea into her arms and she said, "Oh, I need to pray for you! Dear Lord bless this woman and make her well! Heal her Lord! Heal her!Hold her up through her times of suffering! Bless her sweet Lord! Bless this poor woman!"

Cea knew that Sally thought she was me, but she didn't want to interrupt such fine praying and she didn't want to embarrass Sally, so Cea just let Sally whup a healing on her and thanked her very much. Then Cea called me on the phone and told me what happened. We just cracked up. I said, "Why didn't you tell her you were not me?" Cea said, "Are you kidding? I need all the prayers I can get!" So a couple of more weeks went by and I ran into Sally at the assisted living home. When she saw me I said, "Sally, thank you so much for your prayers. I feel good." Sally was grinning from ear to ear and said, "I can tell you feel better. You are sure looking better than the last time I saw you!"

A BREAST NAMED MARILYN MONROE.

Dear Girlfriend,

I went to see my oncologist, Dr. Pippas, after my implant was removed. He looked at the hole in my chest that would not heal and said, "This is horrendous! This is the worst case of radiation damage I have seen in years!" Then he turned to Walker and said, "This is horrendous! Do you know that your wife is going through something horrendous?!" That made me really warm up to Dr. Pippas. He was always very business like and didn't smile very much, which still sort of intimidated me, but when he asked Walker if he knew I was going through something "horrendous" he made me feel like he really cared about me. He didn't say, "Oh, I've seen worse. It's not so bad....." He knew that I was suffering and he didn't trivialize what I was going through. That made me like him very much and raised my respect for him as a physician even more.

There is another physician that works with Dr. Pippas. This doctor has a completely different personality. Where Dr. Pippas is always so serious, Dr. Rodriguez always makes me laugh. Together they really are a dynamic duo. I think of Dr. Pippas as the one who works to heal my body and Dr. Rodriguez is the one who works to heal my troubled mind. After all, laughter is truly healing. Through this whole mess I have tried to rent as many funny movies as I could find and I have tried to hang out with people that are upbeat. Stay away from Gloomy Gus. Gloomy is highly contagious. So on my next trip to the oncologists' office, I first saw Dr. Rodriguez I had told him previously that the casserole brigade had started, so when he came through the door he said, "So, what have the ladies brought you good to eat?"

"Well, we have gotten all kinds of goodies. Cakes... Cookies... all kinds of goodies, but I got out of bed when the pretty little divorcee started e-mailing Walker to check on me. She was too good looking for me to be lying out in the bed looking like death in a pot!"

"Oh, I see. I understand...." Then Dr. Rodriguez took out a notepad and a pen and with a very serious look on his face said, "Okay, now what did you say this beautiful woman's name and phone number are?"

Walker and Dr. Rodriguez and I all just cracked up. It felt so good to laugh with him because it was like being normal again. When you are battling breast cancer, it's easy to just look in the mirror and fall apart. So, when somebody makes you laugh, it's such a gift. It's better than anything you will ever find under the Christmas tree.

Girlfriend advice: Hang out with people who are funny. Spend time with people who make you laugh. I mean this seriously. Laughter is very healing!!!

My breasts were removed in June and the implant was removed in September. Chemotherapy is usually done as soon as the incisions are healed, preferably within six months after the surgery to be the most effective, but I still had a draining hole in my chest that would not close up. Week after week the wound would not heal. Dr. Naman put me on oral antibiotics because the discharge from the wound still showed a low-grade infection. Every day I washed the area around the wound and put petroleum jelly on the skin around it and covered it with sterile gauze. My prosthesis was incredible looking. It looked and felt like a real breast. The problem I had with it was the weight. It weighed about as much as a real breast. If you get a prosthesis after your mastectomy, when you only have a thin, nicely healing incision, then I don't think the weight of it will bother you. However, for me, since I had an open wound, the weight of the prosthesis drove me crazy.

If I wore the prosthesis, I would just slip it into a sports bra because that was so much softer and more comfortable than the regular bras that my insurance had paid for. Anyway I cut the cake, that prosthesis was heavy and totally uncomfortable. I only wore it when I had to leave the house and as soon as I got home, I would run to my bedroom, yank that blankety-blank thing out of my bra, and throw it across the room. Sweet relief! I remember my mother yanking off her girdle when I was a child. Now I could sympathize. I had named my prosthesis Marilyn, after Marilyn Monroe, because it was such a beautiful breast. Walker called it "the titty."

I remember one occasion when I lost "Marilyn." We were getting ready to go out for the evening with some friends. I had thrown Marilyn somewhere and couldn't find her. We had a love-hate relationship you see. I was running all over the house yelling, "Has anybody seen Marilyn!!!???" I had thrown her under the bed or on top of the wardrobe and couldn't find her anywhere. "Walker!!! Have you seen Marilyn!!!??? We're going to be late! Help me find her!" Poor Walker. What that man has had to go through.... So Walker started walking around the house room by room saying, "Here titty! Here titty, titty!"just like he was calling the cat. I said, "If that thing actually comes to you, I'm out of here!" But we did get a good laugh. I told my friend Elaine this story and she told her husband George. Now, every time George loses his car keys he goes around the house hollering, "Here titty! Here titty, titty!" Girlfriend, you have to take a laugh anywhere you can find one.

GOOP + GOOP = GOOP.

Dear Girlfriend,

The weeks just rolled on by and still the hole in my chest would not heal. I have a very dear friend named Josephine. I showed her my chest and she said, "I just can't believe this has happened to you. Your boobs were your calling card. They were famous in Macon! You look like you had a bad ten minutes with a pit bull!" I again appreciated her just telling it like it was instead of saying what most people think they are supposed to say, "Oh, you look fine. Its not so bad!" That response just made me want to say, "Well, if you think this is not so bad, let's just trade breasts. I'll take your lovely breasts and you can take mine, oozy discharge and all."

My friend, Josephine, then moved from one house in our neighborhood to another house in our neighborhood. She decided to have a lady conduct an estate sale in her old house because she was down sizing and did not want to deal with the hassle of selling her own belongings. Now girlfriend, pay close attention to this part of the story because you could blow this off as a coincidence, or you could see the Lord working in mysterious ways through my friend Josephine and her estate sale.

While the sale was going on, Josephine was setting up her furniture and the other items that she had chosen to take with her to her new, smaller house. She was looking around and thought, "I think I can fit that small chair that I left at the old house in that corner. I better drive back over to the old house to get it before it gets sold." So she jumped in her car and drove right back to her old house and ran in the front door to grab the little chair.

When she walked into her old house there were people all over that she did not know. Then a woman who was just about to leave, a woman whom Josephine had never seen before in her life, walked up to her and said, "Is this your house? Are you the one who's having this moving sale?" Josephine said, "Yes, that's me, my name is Josephine." And the woman, I'll call her Cathy said, "My name is Cathy, and I have breast cancer." Now, don't you think this is a little bit weird? I don't remember at any point over the last four years of this mess introducing myself by saying, "Hey! My name is Suzan Rivers and I have breast cancer!" I think that would make people feel very uncomfortable to say the least.

Then Josephine told Cathy, "I have a friend who has breast cancer and she's having a terrible time with radiated skin. The weak skin couldn't hold the implant, so it had to be removed. Now she has been fighting infection for months. No matter what she does, there is a hole in her chest and it just won't heal. They won't let her start chemo until her breast heals completely."

At that Cathy said, "I know what she needs to do." Then Cathy told Josephine the name of a local pharmacist who is very good at compounding various ointments that help skin to heal. Josephine thanked Cathy, grabbed the little chair that she had come after, and drove back to her new house to call me. "Suzan, I've got the name of a local pharmacist who may be able to compound some sort of ointment that will make your breast heal." I was so excited, "Tell me his name and I'll go find him right this minute." She told me his name and the name of the pharmacy. When we hung up I ran to get Walker and told him everything that had just transpired. "Let's go find him right now!" Walker said as we ran out the front door and jumped in the car. "Man, I hope this guy can help you. The months are just rolling by and you really need to get started on that chemotherapy."

When we arrived at the drugstore, we went straight back to the pharmacist. I told him everything that had happened, "I am desperate for you to help me. Do you know of anything that will heal this radiated skin? It's as thin as tissue paper. It couldn't even hold in my implant." The pharmacist was an older gentleman and looked genuinely concerned. He said, "Look, I am so sorry. It's true that I do a lot of compounding, but the compounding I do is from prescriptions that doctors send me. But, I do know a lady that might be able to help you." For one split second I wondered if he were thinking of a conjuror or a root doctor or a faith healer. Lord knows we had tried everything else! And then an angel I'll call Betty finally helped me.

"I want you to go to see this woman who works in our pharmacy warehouse. Her name is Betty. She's the one who fits women with bras and breast prosthesis'. She knows everything there is to know about the healing after mastectomies. Run on over there now before she leaves work."

We thanked him and scooted out to the car. "This is starting to feel like something out of a movie or a scavenger hunt or something," I said. So we rode way out to the other side of town to the pharmacy warehouse. We went inside and found ourselves surrounded by walkers, potty chairs, wheelchairs and the like. We went to the counter and I asked, "Where would I find a lady named Betty?" The man behind the counter said, "She's in that room at the back of the warehouse. Just go knock on her door." Walker stayed up front while I walked through rows of medical equipment to get to Betty's office. I knocked on the door and she opened it.

"Are you Betty?"

"Yes, ma'am. That's me. How can I help you?" I sat down and proceeded to tell her my whole story. "So, you're just having a bad time of it?" she said.

"I am totally desperate. I need for my chest to heal so I can start chemotherapy." I lamented. "Well honey, I'll have to have a look at your wound," she said and I began taking my shirt and bra off for yet another stranger. She looked at my chest and said, "Bless your heart. I think you breast cancer ladies are so strong. I can tell by looking that you've had a horrible time."

"Have you got any suggestions?"

"Well, darlin', here's the thing. You've got goop."

I was very aware of the light colored green goop that filled the hole in my chest. "Can you get rid of it?"

"Well, now, tell me what you're doing to heal this wound?"

"I clean it everyday, and then I put petroleum jelly around it and cover it with gauze."

"Well, that's the problem. You want to get rid of the goop, but you're just adding more goop by putting petroleum jelly on it. We want this hole to dry up. It won't ever dry up the way you're treating it." Then she sat down on a chair next to me and spoke to me like I was a little child or maybe just stupid. She leaned forward and looked me square in the eyes. "Honey, you've got goop. Goop plus goop equals?"

I took a guess and said, "More goop?"

She leaned back on her chair, slapped both knees with her hands and said, "That's right!" I felt like an idiot, but there was just something about her that I liked so much. Then she said, "Look here. I'm no doctor and I'm no nurse, so you aren't gonna come back and sue me are you?"

"Oh no ma'am! I would never do that. I would just be so grateful if you can tell me how to heal this wound."

"Okay, what we're gonna do is dry the wound out. We're gonna stop putting any petroleum jelly or any other kind of oil on it. First, I want you to buy some saline solution. We sell it right here. Spray it twice a day with that saline solution. Do you remember when you were a little girl and you went to the beach, and if you had any kind of cut or scrape, the salt water would heal you?"

"I do remember that."

"Well, I'm going to treat you just like you were at the beach. Salt water and seaweed."

"Seaweed? I don't think my doctor will let me put seaweed on my chest...."

"Honey, I'm gonna use a special gauze that's made out of seaweed." She went to her cabinet of medical supplies and took out a packet. Inside the packet was a single piece of sterile white gauze, that looked exactly like any other piece of white gauze that I had ever seen. "Now, if you spray that wound with saline solution and then lay a piece of this 'Aquacel' gauze over the wound, that gauze will pull all of that mess out of your wound and your wound will just dry up and heal. It works every time."

That made perfect sense. The next day I took the gauze to Dr. Naman, my plastic surgeon. Then I took it to my oncologist, Dr. Pippas. Both of them thought that using the 'Aquacel' was a good idea. Walker ordered a supply of it off the internet for one third of what it cost at the drugstore. I did exactly like Betty instructed. I sprayed the wound with saline solution, dried it very gently with a clean towel, and then laid the 'Aquacel' over the wound. I used a cloth tape to hold it in place. It started working almost immediately. The goop just dried up and the skin closed up almost completely.

I was healed. Now, you can just believe that all this was a series of coincidences, but I choose to believe that God had a hand in this. What was the chance that my friend Josephine entered her old residence at the very second Cathy was about to leave? What compelled Cathy, to tell a total stranger, Josephine, that she had breast cancer? What compelled Josephine to call me and tell me what Cathy had told her? What compelled the pharmacist to direct me to Betty at the warehouse? And what compelled Betty to help me? It is possible that all of this was just a series of coincidences, but I prayed for that hole in my chest to heal, and other than popping up and laying his hands on me, how was God supposed to make that happen? It happened in a way that I could understand. God puts the power of knowing what to do into people, so that they can carry out His work of healing the sick.

You see, if any one step in this chain of events had not played out the exact way it did, then there is no telling how long I would have had to wait for my wound to heal. As it happened, I was able to start my chemotherapy in November, five months after my bilateral mastectomy was performed. Yes, the Lord does work in mysterious ways.

Girlfriend advice: Before you start radiation, make positively sure that your radiation oncologist is going to use the most up to date, state of the art equipment and procedures. Get on the internet and research this thoroughly. Research this before you let any physician do radiation on your breast. Radiation can be a tool of healing, but it can also do great damage to your delicate body.

I had external radiation. Research internal radiation which is called bracytherapy. This type of radiation uses tiny radioactive pellets that are placed inside the breast. An excellent website to research bracytherapy is www.arizonabreastcancerspecialists.com. Go to the finest facility that your insurance allows. There is nothing wrong with asking questions about the procedures and equipment that your doctor plans to use. Make sure you are convinced that you are getting the best treatment possible.

FEAR OF CHEMO. I WAS SO ANGRY AT GOD.

Dear Girlfriend,

My breasts were removed in June, 2010. My chemotherapy could not start until November, 2010, when my open wound finally closed up. That meant that I had five long months for my fear of chemo to get ramped up. This fear had an awful lot to do with the fact that all five of my girlfriends who had died of cancer the year before, were doing chemo when they died. Now, let me stop right here. All five of my friends that died of various kinds of cancer were already Stage Four when their cancer was discovered. That means that their cancer had already spread throughout their bodies before they began chemotherapy. But, in my mind, I associated chemotherapy with loved ones dying. I thought of chemotherapy as something to fear and something to dread, not as something wonderful that could save my life. Girlfriend, I was terrified that something would go wrong and I would not survive chemo.

After all, look at everything that had already gone wrong. My cancer that was not supposed to come back had indeed come back. I had developed a horrible staph infection. My implant had ripped out four times and had to be removed because the radiation had made my skin too weak to hold the implant. My skin damaged by radiation left a hole in my chest that oozed goop for five months before it healed. So, yes, I was terrified that something else would go wrong if I did chemotherapy.

I remember that my girlfriend, Janet, had encouraged me months before to get on Facebook. I have never been very fond of computers and I rarely take photographs, but she said one day when she was visiting me at "Fairy Ring Cottage", our cottage in the woods, "Give me your computer. I'm going to put you on Facebook. Everybody wants to keep up with what's going on with you. You're going to love it!" So, I got on Facebook and started to give my "Friends" the update on what was happening with me. I was totally blown away by the outpouring of love that came to me from people on Facebook.

As the day for my chemo approached, I became more and more afraid. With my track record of things going wrong, you can see why I was almost out of my mind with fear. Dr. Pippas sent me to an orientation to chemotherapy with some other cancer patients. There I learned what chemo does and how it works. Chemotherapy is generally used when breast cancer has gone to the lymph nodes. Although I had just a microscopic metastasis, I had a recurrence in less than a year, so Dr. Pippas thought it best that I do chemo.

So what is chemotherapy? Well, girlfriend, this is where you need to have your doctor sit down and explain, in terms you can understand, just exactly what your chemo regimen will be. After all, I am not a doctor, I am writing this book to help you survive the damage that cancer can reek on you physically, mentally and spiritually. I am writing to tell you how to find inner peace. But I am not qualified to tell you all that you need to know about how cancer and chemo actually work. Please go to your doctor for an expert medical explanation. Now I'll tell you how I came to think of cancer and chemotherapy in my "not a physician's brain."

You have millions of cells in your body. You have millions of cells in your breast. When cells are doing what they are supposed to do, they replicate. That means that they make other cells just like themselves. Every cell in your breast, every cell in your body goes through phases. In the first phase, the cell does nothing. In the next phase, if the cell is doing what it is supposed to do, it divides and creates another cell just like the original cell. This cell division, one cell dividing into two cells, is called mitosis. Yep, that stuff you had to learn in high school biology class is starting to take on some real meaning now! And you wondered why you had to learn all that boring stuff. Now that we're talking about saving your life, it's not boring anymore....

So to make a long story short, if your breast cells are behaving themselves, they are making new cells that are just like the old ones. When your breast cells start making cells that are not just like the old ones, they are mutated cells. I think of them as gangsters. When all these bad guys, these mutated cells, start hanging out together in a bunch, you have a tumor. And just like a bunch of gangsters hanging out together, a tumor is going to cause trouble. There are several ways to deal with a tumor. You can just cut it out, a lumpectomy. You can cut it out and do radiation on the area where the tumor was to try to make sure all the "gangster" cells in the surrounding area are zapped. But, look at me. I had a lumpectomy and radiation and those little cancer cells came right on back in just one year. So how do you know if you for absolutely sure got rid of every single cancer cell in your body? You don't know.

That is what is hard about having cancer. You can't ever be absolutely sure that you got all of those cancer cells. Chemotherapy is just pulling out the biggest, baddest guns to do all that is possible to get all those gangster cells throughout your whole body. Chemotherapy is used to kill those slippery little suckers that may have escaped the surgeon's knife and the power of radiation. I guess when it comes down to it you are doing battle with yourself.

That sounds pretty weird doesn't it? When you have cancer, you really do come to the reality that you are a duel being. Your physical self is trying to commit suicide without the permission of your mental and spiritual self. And when you realize that that is really what is going on, then you come to a whole deeper understanding of what it means to be a human being. You want to live! You want your cells to behave themselves so that your physical body can be healthy. You want to be around to see your children's children's children. Or maybe you were getting close to getting that big promotion or you were going to be president of the company. You finally got your ducks in a row to buy your dream house or your wedding day was only six weeks away... and then you find a lump.

Then your entire game plan changes overnight. The only thing you can focus on is doing battle with your own body, because like I said before, you come to the realization that you are not in control of what happens in your body. You are on automatic. You don't have control over your cell replication. God does. You might have the power to be the CEO of a big corporation, but you can't even make your own cells behave themselves.

When you get down to it, "powerful" is not an adjective that should ever be used to describe a human being. You can't even control the inner workings of your own body. You might be the next president of the United States, but you are not powerful. Your cells have gone gangster, your own cells are trying to kill you. So now your only option is to hand over your mind and soul to God, so that He can show you the way to be healed. Let God infiltrate your mind and your soul to save your physical self. Think of yourself as going to war. What are you going to use to kill the enemy, Cancer?

Think again of David getting ready to do battle with Goliath. David had to look and choose just the right rocks to use in his slingshot to kill the giant Goliath. Do you think he picked up a few little pebbles? Heck no! He scrambled around as fast as he could and chose some big ole rocks that could kill that giant before that giant killed him. And you have to do the same thing if you are going to survive cancer. You and your doctor have to make a battle plan.

The first phase of my battle plan didn't work. The first phase was a lumpectomy, radiation and Tamoxifen. After one year my cancer came back and so my surgeon and I decided that both of my breasts should be removed and my oncologist told me that he thought I should do chemo. Now I could have refused, but like David, I picked up the biggest rocks I could find to kill my opponent, Cancer. Dr. Pippas decided to use four doses of Taxotere and Cytoxan given to me through my port once every three weeks. That meant a total of four treatments in twelve weeks.

This chemo regimen is called systemic treatment because it aims to kill cancer cells throughout the entire body. Chemotherapy drugs attack cancer cells and take away their ability to replicate and so they die. Bombs away! The problem is that, as in any war, some of the good guy cells are killed too. These can be in your hair follicles, mouth, vagina, bone marrow and intestines. Chemotherapy attacks cells that divide rapidly. Cancer cells divide rapidly so chemo targets those cells. The cells in your hair follicles divide rapidly, so they get it too, and that's why the hair falls out.

Dr. Pippas also had me take a shot of Neulasta the day after receiving each of my infusions of chemo in order to pump up my white cell count. Remember, those white cells are the soldier cells that fight all sorts of infections, so you want to keep a good white cell count while you are doing chemotherapy. So my first chemo infusion was scheduled in November, right around Thanksgiving. As the day drew closer, the more afraid I became. Walker and I drove from our house in Macon to Fairy Ring Cottage the day before my treatment because the cottage, way back in the forest on Pine Mountain, is just a thirty minute drive to Columbus, where I was scheduled for my first infusion.

Now, remember what I told you. Having cancer is like your own physical body deciding to self destruct without your permission. So, you have to use your mind, and the minds of your doctors, to out smart your body which has decided to go haywire on a cellular level. But like I said before, you are a duel being. Your mind is actually part of your physical being, you can use your mind to decide what treatments you will use to fight that part of your body that has gone the way of cancer. Your physical self includes your brain, which controls your thoughts, but your spirit or soul is that part of you that never dies. You must be totally willing for God, your Creator, to take control of your mind and your soul in order for you to accept whatever God has planned for you. When you can get to the point where you can trust God's plan for you, whether it is to live on earth in your physical body until you are one hundred or only thirty, then you are truly at peace. You realize that it doesn't really matter how long you stay here on Earth in your physical and mental body because your spirit will live forever.

And girlfriend, I can tell you that I was not at the stage of trusting in God's plan for me when the day before my first chemo infusion arrived. Walker and I got to the cottage and as soon as the sun went down, I started to cry. I was terrified that something terrible would go wrong and my physical body would die. I was not yet ready to give up my fear of physical death. I was flat freaking out. I remember that I went into the bathroom and took off all of my clothes and just looked at my body in the mirror. Having only one breast had already gone on for five months. I still looked pale and white and hideous. I got in the bathtub and just cried and cried and then for the first time since I was diagnosed, I got mad.

I was mad at God. I was mad that God was allowing me to go through all this suffering. I remember for the first time in my life, I sat in that bathtub with tears rolling down my face and I looked up to heaven, and I shook my fist at God. I shook my fist in sheer anger, the deepest rage I had ever felt.

I said, "God! I don't understand you!!! You are supposed to be all loving. You are supposed to be all powerful! I am supposed to be your child! If you love me and you have the power to cure me and save me from all this suffering, then why don't you just do it?! I am nothing but a lowly human being, but I can tell you one thing God, if one of my children had cancer and I had the power to just instantly heal her, I WOULD HEAL HER!!! And God, if I had the power to heal her and take away all her suffering and I CHOSE not to heal her, that would be a grave, dark, mortal sin!!! If I had the power to cure her and stop her suffering and just decided to let her keep on suffering, I would be the worst mother in the world!!! So God, how can you call yourself all loving, when you know you have the power to heal me instantly and instead you are just letting my suffering continue on and on and on???!!! So what makes you such an all good and all loving God???!!!"

I guess He could have struck me down with a thunderbolt, but He didn't. He didn't smite me or smote me or whatever that word is that means zapped. Then I got out of the bathtub and went to my computer. I wrote on Facebook that I was terrified and I asked all my friends to pray that I would stop feeling afraid. I asked my friends to pray that I would find the courage to get up in the morning and head to Columbus to take that chemotherapy. Then I just went to bed, curled up in Walker's arms and cried myself to sleep. As I drifted off I heard him say, "I love you, Boo Boo..."

When I woke up the next morning, Walker was standing over me with a cup of coffee. "Hey, Suzy-Q, you need to get up. You've got to get ready to go to Columbus," he said with a wary look on his face. I think he was expecting me to jump up and scoot under the bed to hide. Much to his surprise I just calmly sat up, took the coffee from him and said, "Okay. Thank you." Girlfriend, I was totally peaceful and unafraid. All those friends on Facebook had prayed for me to be at peace and I woke up in a totally tranquil mood. Unsmited. Unsmoted. I sat in bed and drank my coffee and remembered to put on my Lidocaine ointment that I had left out on my bedside table. Remember, Lidocaine is a numbing cream. I put a generous amount on the area of my chest where my chemo port had been inserted. Then I just got up and put on my soft comfy cotton knit dress and a warm snuggy sweater and walked downstairs. Walker was still waiting for me to go into freak -out mode, but I didn't.

MY FIRST CHEMO. I AM LIKE THE BUG ON THE CEILING.

Dear Girlfriend,

We got in the car and drove on down to Columbus. We walked into the John B. Amos Cancer Center and were directed to the infusion center. I was completely calm. I know Walker must have thought aliens from space had come in the night and taken over my body, or something, because I was calm and smiling and cheerful. The power of prayer, you just can't beat it....

I didn't really know what to expect, but going into the infusion center was not scary. The room was full of cozy recliner chairs. Everyone in there was laid back reading books, eating snacks, or working on laptops. A few people had their eyes closed so I guess they were asleep. Most of the patients had one friend or one relative sitting beside them. Some of these people were talking to their chemo buddies and some were watching TV together and not talking.

Walker and I were escorted over to a recliner by a friendly young female nurse. "Mrs. Rivers, did you remember to put some numbing cream on your port?" she asked. "Yes, I did," I replied. "Well then, just make yourself comfortable in this chair while I go get you some nice warmed up blankets. We have a blanket warmer and everybody loves those warmed up blankets." She walked away and I sat in the recliner. Walker sat down in the "buddy" chair right next to me. In a minute the nurse came back with some toasty warm blankies and tucked me into the chair.

"Are you alright? Are you nervous?" she asked. "I might be getting a little nervous," I said. "Well, I put something in your bag that will take away that nervous feeling." Then she cleaned the area over my port, dried off the area and inserted a needle into the port right through my skin. Since I had numbed up the area with Lidocaine, I didn't feel any pain at all. What a relief! Then she attached the needle to a tube that was attached to my bag of chemo drugs and my "happy" drug.

"Are you comfortable? Can I get you a soft drink or crackers, juice, yogurt, pudding? Anything?" she asked. That happy medicine was already starting to take effect, so I just settled back and said, "I'm fine. Just fine." She smiled and said, "Okay, you just stay put and our dietician is going to come talk to you in a minute." I was starting to feel pleasantly woozy when a very friendly lady approached my chair. "Hello. I'm Beth. I'm the dietician. Would it be alright if I visit with you a little while?" We introduced ourselves and she pulled up a chair to talk to Walker and me. She said that usually on the day that a patient receives a chemotherapy infusion, they feel just fine, but on the next day or the third day I might feel nauseated and lose my appetite. She told me that Dr. Pippas had prescribed a wonderful anti-nausea drug for me. This drug is called Zofran and it is so effective that some people call it Saint Zofran.

I was listening to everything she said, but Saint Happy Drug was making me a little sleepy. Walker was, as always, listening to every word she said and taking notes. She was all about preventing my breast cancer from coming back, by getting me into an anti- cancer lifestyle. We talked about what causes breast cancer. From all the research that has been done there are quite a few things that doctors believe contribute to getting breast cancer.

Using hormone replacement therapy, HRT, can increase the risk of breast cancer in some women. It had already been determined that my body's reaction to estrogen was not a good one. Being overweight and lack of exercise can increase your risk of development of breast cancer. Having more than one serving of alcohol a day significantly raises the risk of breast cancer. Having close relatives who have had breast cancer can increase your risk.

But, since I already had breast cancer, Beth turned the conversation towards preventing another recurrence. "You really can decrease your chances of breast cancer with your diet. You need to eat lots of dark leafy green vegetables like cabbage and Brussels sprouts. I want you to eat blueberries, dark purple grapes and stone fruits."

"What are stone fruits? I asked.

"Stone fruits are fruits that have large pits in them like peaches, plums and mangoes."

"Is there anything else I can do to keep from getting cancer again?"

"Yes. Take calcium citrate with Vitamin D. This is really important. Don't take calcium carbonate because it's made from ground up oyster shells and can cause kidney stones. Make sure it is calcium citrate with Vitamin D for the best absorption. I also want you to take fish oil. It comes in a gel cap so you don't have to taste it, and if you get enteric coated fish oil capsules you won't have fish burps or indigestion,"she said.

"Is there anything else?" I asked. " Take a good multiple vitamin daily, avoid white refined sugar as much as possible. Eat garlic. Garlic is a real anti-cancer food. Just live a good healthy lifestyle. Eat your fruits and veggies, keep your weight down, exercise.

Eat ground golden flaxseed. Ground flaxseed blocks the effects of natural estrogen on cells. Since your cancer was estrogen driven, ground flaxseed might just be good protection against a recurrence of your cancer. It's great in smoothies. You can put blueberries, peaches, ground golden flaxseed and lowfat organic milk and blend them up together. It really tastes good and just might decrease your chances of a recurrence. You can actually buy a little smoothie maker that mixes up your smoothie right in the glass you'll drink it from. I like mine a lot because it's so easy to wash. I hate the hassle of having to wash a big blender for one little smoothie."

"Well, what do you mean by organic milk?" I asked.

"I mean milk that comes from cows that were not shot full of hormones. You really should stick to meats and eggs that come from animals that were not shot up with hormones. You need to stay away from estrogen. Estrogen can act like fertilizer to breast cancer cells."

"What can she eat while she's on chemotherapy? Walker asked.

"She can eat anything she feels like eating, but most people do well with ice cream and pudding, cold foods, light foods. It just depends on how she feels."

"Can you think of some more things I can do to prevent another recurrence?" I asked.

"Well, use deodorant that doesn't have aluminum in it. Don't even cook in aluminum pots. Don't use cookware that has the nonstick surface worn off. Cook in glass, stainless steel or cast iron. And don't heat up your food in the microwave in plastic. Heat up your food in glass. If you have any questions just call me. Here's my phone number...."

After Beth left, I stayed in the recliner about another hour. Walker was working on his laptop while I just sort of floated away with my Saint Happy Drug that was going into my body along with an anti- nausea drug and the chemo medicine. I was trying to visualize the chemo pouring into my veins like little PacMan creatures finding the cancer cells and gobbling them up. The time passed quickly and the sweet nurse who had hooked me up to the chemo bag came back to unhook me. "So how do you feel? Are you okay?" I felt pleasantly drugged, just a little bit sleepy.... "I'm fine," I said as she took the needle out of my port and helped me out of the recliner.

"Now, don't forget that you have to come back in the morning to get your Neulasta shot. We have to keep those white blood cells pumped up so you won't get any infections. Try to avoid going out in crowds where people will be coughing and sneezing around you and don't be hugging a lot of people through the holidays. Your immune system is going to be compromised and you have to think about staying well. Even a cold can make you feel really sick when you're on chemo," she said. "Well, I got a flu shot about a month ago," I told her. "That was a good idea. The flu can knock you down pretty hard when you're doing chemo."

After I was all unhooked we left the center, got in the car and drove back to Fairy Ring Cottage. I was waiting to see what was going to happen. I was waiting to see if I got deathly sick. I felt just fine in the car. When we got to the cottage, Walker built a cozy fire in the fireplace and turned on the lights on our little bitty baby Christmas tree. I must admit it had been a good day. All that crying and carrying on for nothing.... "How do you feel?" Walker asked as we snuggled up together under a blanket by the fireplace. "I feel just fine," I said as I lay my head on his shoulder....

In awhile he got up to fix himself a snack and I stretched out on the couch. I was just looking up at the ceiling and I noticed a little bug crawling around up there. He was obviously lost. He was just wandering around this way and that way trying to find a way to get back outside. From my perspective I could see that all he needed to do was crawl over to the crack in the door and go right on out. But, Mr. Bug could not see the whole picture. He could only see what was right in front of him. His vision of the situation was so limited that he had no idea of the reality of the total situation in which he found himself.

Then it hit me. I was like the bug. You are like the bug. Every human being on this planet is just like the bug. A couple of nights before I had cried and railed against God, "If you are a loving God, why are you allowing me to suffer so much? Why don't you just make this suffering stop right now? If you love me why don't you heal me instantly?!" I cried out to God. I got no answer, just silence. Now I could see the answer. We, as humans, just like the bug, can't see the entire picture. God can see the entire picture. He sees me suffer and he doesn't heal me instantly. He sees some people suffer and does not heal them at all. And we think why? Why does he allow sickness and suffering? The only thing I came up with is that God can see the total picture and we can't.

God looks at the whole picture and sees that our human suffering, in some way, somehow, is for good. Just like when a mother is in labor. She suffers through a great deal of pain, but in the end she has the joy of a having a new baby. Suffering is part of this life on earth. Cancer causes us to suffer, but God in some mysterious way uses our suffering for good. I have to believe that is true in order to stay happy in this life. I am like the bug on the ceiling. I can't see where I am going. I have no idea where I am, out here in the cosmos on a rock that is spinning around a great ball of fire. I am surrounded by billions and billions of other spinning rocks and balls of fire that go on and on infinitely.... Why am I here in this strange place, in this strange situation? All I can do is have faith that there is a loving God that knows why I am here, and He is using my suffering for the greater good that is his plan for this universe. I hope that when I go to heaven God will let me see the total picture. I hope that He will say, "Look, I created this universe and allowed it to become what it has become. In order for it to become what it has become there was great suffering all along the way, but see my creation is good. Your suffering contributed to that good." That would be heaven to me, just knowing that human suffering, in the end, contributed to a good creation.

The next morning we were up and out on the road to the infusion center again to get the Neulasta shot. I had a male nurse this time and it was no big deal. No pain. Use Lidocaine! After receiving the shot we drove on back to Macon. That day passed and the next day too, but I really felt fine. On the third day I noticed that anything and everything I tried to eat tasted peculiar. It tasted like metal. I had been taking my Zofran three times a day, even though I had not experienced any nausea. Dr. Pippas had told me to stay one step ahead of the nausea. Girlfriend, I think that was some very important advice. I took Zofran every single day for the next three weeks and I never experienced any nausea. Good ole Dr. Pippas for prescribing Zofran the "wonder drug". I did have some very bad indigestion that made me start to cough. I remember coughing so hard that I did actually throw up, but I was not nauseated one time during the whole three week period.

> **Girlfriend advice: Take your prescribed nausea medication before you ever get nauseated the first time. There may be some other brands out there that work, but I'm telling you, Zofran worked very very well for me. You might want to ask your doctor about it! If you keep taking your nausea medication you might get lucky like I did and never get nauseated the first time.**

GOING BALD. MAMA, YOU LOOK LIKE BENJAMIN FRANKLIN.

Dear Girlfriend,

I went on with life as usual because Christmas time had rolled around again. I had to do all my shopping and wrapping presents, decorating, cooking, etc., while I was doing chemo. Like I told you in the beginning, cancer does not give you any time out. Everybody still expects you to do what you always have done before, even if you are doing chemo, and you will not want to disappoint them.

Right before Christmas, 2008, I was diagnosed with cancer. The next Christmas, 2009, I had already had the lumpectomy, radiation and was taking Tamoxifen. I thought I was cured so we had a very good Christmas that year. Unfortunately, my cancer came back. The year 2010 was filled with that heart wrenching news, the bilateral mastectomy, the staph infection, the implant ripping out and being removed , the hole in my chest that took five months to heal and now chemotherapy. What next? Thank God the we can't see too far down the road....

A few days passed and I woke up with my entire scalp slightly aching. I didn't know that that was a sign that my hair was about to fall out. As the day wore on, I realized that if I pulled on my hair ever so slightly, a few strands of hair would just come right out. But, it was two weeks until Christmas and I had major shopping that I still had to get done.

Everybody wanted to keep up with my treatment on Facebook so I posted this:

"Today my hair started to fall out. I'm afraid I'm going to look like one of those Sea Monkeys that you could order out of the back of comic books when I was a kid. You were supposed to just drop the magic tablets in water and the sea monkeys would grow. The picture in the comic books was of this creature with huge eyes and a big bald head. I'm afraid that's going to be the new me."

So even though I knew my hair was about to all fall out, I just absolutely had to get my Christmas shopping done. Mama makes the magic. You know exactly what I'm talking about. I didn't have the luxury of sitting around feeling sorry for myself, I had to pull off Christmas. So I went to Barnes and Noble and ran into a friend of mine. My hair, at that point, didn't really look much different because I was so careful not to touch it. If I tried to brush it or tug on it ever so slightly, out it came. But, it didn't hurt at all. You would think that it would hurt to pull it out, but it didn't hurt one little bit.

So, when I ran into my friend, Cindy, at Barnes and Noble she said, "Now, I don't believe what you put on Facebook, your hair looks just fine!" At that I just reached up and pulled a glob of hair right out of my head. "Oh my God! I believe you!" she said as she grabbed the hair out of my hand and crammed it down into her empty paper coffee cup that she was about to throw away. We didn't know what else to say so we just busted out laughing. The whole scene was just crazy. I spent the rest of the day doing as much shopping as I could because I knew that the big event was about to happen, and I wasn't sure if I was going to be in the Christmas spirit after going completely bald.

The next day I woke up with my scalp really aching badly. On the day your hair falls out, your whole scalp really aches. Before I had a chance to let that little reality set in, I also discovered what every woman knows is the worst thing ever... I had a bladder infection. I barely made it out of bed and into the bathroom before the urine, which felt like burning liquid fire, started to come out of me, as you well know, three drops at a time.... So, there I was, sitting on the potty, in complete misery when I unthinkingly ran my hand up through my hair and a huge wad just came out in my hand. I thought I would die. I managed to get to the medicine cabinet and thank God I had a bottle of Pyridium to stop the burning sensation when I urinated. What a mess!!! I was unable to get five feet away from the toilet without having to go again, and my hair was just coming out in big wads if I just touched it at all.

I called Lori, my nurse navigator, and told her what was going on. "When you're doing chemo, it's common to come down with all kinds of infections. I'll call some antibiotics in to your pharmacy. I know you're upset about your hair...." At that point I was just about in tears. Lori added, "This is just going to be a hard day. I'll phone you in some Xanax to calm you down. Oh, and don't shave your head, I don't want to risk your cutting yourself and getting another infection. You can just brush your hair out with a clean hairbrush."

So wasn't I just in a pretty fix? Sitting on the potty while liquid fire dripped and my hair doing the grand finale act of all falling out. Girlfriend, I never in my life dreamed that I would have to go through something this awful. But, whatever happens to you, hold onto the thought that it is only temporary. You can make it! I wish someone had kept on telling me that. I just remember waiting and praying that the Pyridium would take effect and stop the burning, at least long enough for me to get to my grocery store pharmacy to get the Xanax before I had a complete nervous breakdown. And let me add right here that mothers at Christmas are not allowed to have nervous breakdowns!!!

So, I just sat there until the burning sensation stopped and then I headed for the grocery store to get my prescription for Xanax filled. When I got inside the grocery store, I ran into another friend, like I had run into Cindy at Barnes and Noble. What was so funny to me was the exact same scene was played out all over again. This time it was Julie who said, "Suzan, your hair looks fine!" At that I just ran my hand through my hair and another big glob came out. Julie reacted the exact same way that Cindy had reacted. She said, "Oh my God!" as she grabbed the hair out of my hand and quickly stuffed it down in her pocketbook. Then we both just cracked up. What else could we do?

I don't know why both Cindy and Julie felt compelled to grab my hair and hide it, but that must be the proper etiquette for the situation because that's what both of them did. So I went on over and got in line to pick up my prescription that Lori had called in from Dr. Pippas's office in Columbus. The line was long. Very long. As I stood there, I realized that everybody in line was coughing and sneezing all over me. I kept thinking,

"Yikes! I've got to get out of here before I catch the bubonic plague!" I stood in that line over a half hour. When I finally got up to the counter, I told the girl that I needed to pick up my prescription for Xanax, which had been called in from Columbus. Then she said ,"I'm sorry, but I can't fill anymore prescriptions today because our server just went down."

At that point I had just about had enough. I said, "Look, I'm on chemo and my hair is falling out today. By this evening I'll be completely bald and this has gotten me very upset!!!" At that I reached up and yanked a huge glob of my hair out right off the top of my head. I just stood there holding that big glob of hair in my hand and said, " I really NEED that Xanax!!!" Well, girlfriend, I have good news to share, prescriptions can still be filled even when "the server has gone down." You have never seen anybody put pills in a bottle faster than that poor girl did. I guess she thought I was going to blow up the grocery store, or at the very least take out a gun and shoot her.

I looked at the people who were standing in line behind me and all of their mouths were just hanging wide open. One lady understood what had just transpired and she said, "Don't you worry, honey, I've been through it myself. You're going to be just fine. You're just having a bad hair day!"

I think that was an understatement. Losing my hair was making me wig out! I got my Xanax and antibiotics and drove on back to the house. I took a Xanax and tried to calm down. I went and got the wig that I had bought ahead of time, at the breast cancer boutique, for this special occasion. After awhile I felt alright. Better living through chemicals....

I decided that I needed to get rid of all the rest of my hair before I scared somebody else. I called two of my college-aged daughters into the bathroom to help me. "Okay girls, we're just going to take these two new hairbrushes and brush all of the hair out," I said.

My daughter Laurel immediately sat on the floor in the lotus position and started to meditate, "Oooooommmmm."

I said, "What in the world are you doing?"

"Oh Mama, I'm going to have to go to therapy after this!" she replied.

My other daughter, Blythe, just sat quietly on the side of the bathtub. I starting brushing and singing the theme to Hair. Blythe took up the other brush and together we just kept on brushing and brushing while the hair fell out all over me and all over the bathroom floor. At first I looked like a moth eaten sweater. Then in a little while Laurel just started laughing. Blythe had not said word one through this whole drama, but I could tell she was trying hard not to laugh. Laurel was laughing hysterically. So I said, "What's the matter with you? Laughing at your poor little Mama losing all her hair?"

Laurel said, "Mama, look in the mirror. You look just like Benjamin Franklin!!!"

It was so true. All the hair on the top of my head and about half way down was gone, but the rest of my hair was straggling down to my shoulders. "You know what? You're right. I do look like Benjamin Franklin. All I need is a pair of those natty little spectacles...." Then all three of us just howled. Blythe and I continued to brush until Benjamin was gone. Wow... what a shock.... Finally I said to Laurel, "Why are we laughing? I look like hell!!!" Laurel said, "I think this is like when people laugh at funeral receptions. They laugh to keep from crying." What she said was true, and I realized how grown up both of my college girls were by the way they helped me that day.

Then Blythe just took the wig and placed it on my head. Laurel said, "Let's call her Foxy." So I had a fake breast named "Marilyn" and a wig named "Foxy." I looked in the mirror to see if there was any "Suzan" left. Blythe brushed "Foxy" out all nice and pretty and Laurel handed me some long, dangly, sparkly earrings. I put on the earrings, stared at the new me in the mirror and said, "Cancer, go jump! We're having fun with this...." Thank the Lord for daughters....

> **Girlfriend advice: Before you start chemo, have your doctor prescribe Pyridium just in case you get a bladder infection. Think ahead and talk to your doctor about meds you should have on hand to make chemotherapy a lot easier. Buy your synthetic wig before your hair falls out. Practice wearing it before the blessed event happens so you will feel more comfortable with your new hot look!**

I HAVE A FLAT HEAD.

Dear Girlfriend,

Walker and I returned to the chemo infusion center for my second infusion on December 20, 2010, just five days before Christmas. So far I had done very well with chemotherapy. Food tasted awful, but I was eating a little and drinking lots of fluids even though I had no appetite. I knew I needed to eat in order to stay strong and fight infection. On my second infusion I got all bundled up in my recliner, hooked up to the medication bag and just relaxed. "Walker, you don't have to stay with me. I'm fine. You should go visit your mother until I'm finished," I said. "Are you sure?" he asked. "I'm just fine. Go take a break."

He left and I just sat back and messed around on my laptop. I was very calm. I was not in any pain. The only bad part of the experience was looking around at some of the other patients. Most of them looked well enough, but some of them did look very sick. I felt so sorry for them and I said prayers for each one of them. I noticed that several of the women were wearing little knit caps and scarves and I was wearing Foxy. The anticipation of losing my hair had been torture to me. The thought of going bald had been absolutely awful. When my hair actually fell out, the event wasn't as bad as I had thought it would be. Going through the chemo infusions was not as bad as I thought it would be. I made it through my second chemo infusion just fine. What was difficult for me was the way being bald and having only one breast made me feel so utterly unattractive.

The day I lost my hair was December 16, 2010. My second chemo infusion was December 20, 2010. I guess you are wondering how you are supposed to keep an intimate relationship going when you are bald and only have one breast. Did I feel pretty? No. Did I feel sexy? No. I felt gross and hideous. I'm not going to sit here and lie to you. I felt like I was absolutely disgusting. A friend of mine gave me a darling little hat. When I put it on I looked like Charlie Chaplin. Another friend gave me a beautiful silk scarf. When I put it on I looked like a gypsy fortune teller. All I needed to do was hang out a sign, "Sister Suzan Sees All." I lost every single bit of hair on my entire body. Yep. There too.

Needless to say, sex was not even on my mind. I still liked for Walker to hold me, but that was about it. I tried very hard to not let him see me without a shirt on. I wore pretty nightgowns or a nice camisole to bed. Some women feel comfortable with their lover seeing them without a breast, but I did not. I stayed covered up as much as possible. I really didn't feel comfortable walking around the house bald. If you feel okay with that, then more power to you! If I had a beautifully shaped head, I might have felt differently, but my head turned out to be as flat as a runway in the back.

"See how flat my head is? Now you can't ever get mad at me again for not being able to read a map! I told you there had to be some reason I can't do math and have no sense of time or direction. See Walker! Just look at this flat head! My mother must have dropped me or something...."

"I thought you said you couldn't do all those things because you had a fever that was so high you had to be hospitalized when you were three years old," he replied.

"Well, I'm sure that was part of the problem, too, but just look at this flat head. Maybe my mother never picked me up when I was a baby, and that made my head flat and squished out most of my smarts. Just think what I could have been if I hadn't been brain squished!" Walker just rolled his eyes and shook his head as usual.

Since my head did not have a pretty shape I never went around the house bald.

I wore Foxy when I had to leave the house and I wore my "Anne Boleyn is about to get her head chopped off cap" when I was at home. I even wore the cap to bed. I called it my "Anne Boleyn is about to get her head chopped off cap" because we had just recently watched a movie on television about Henry VIII and his six wives. Before Anne Boleyn got her head chopped off, she put on a little skull cap that looked very similar to mine. So now I had "Marilyn", the perfect breast, "Foxy" the wig and a cap that was named my "Ann Boleyn's about to get her head chopped off cap."

One day Walker said, "You know Boo Boo, if you ever decide to start marketing those caps yourself, you might want to consider changing the name of the cap."

"I'll take your suggestion into consideration," I replied.

There was something I noticed about being bald in winter. Even with my cap, my head stayed cold. You know that line in *The Night Before Christmas*, "Ma in her kerchief and I in my cap, had just settled down for a long winter's nap...." Now, I have a whole new understanding of that line. People wore caps to bed in the old days because their houses were so cold that their heads were freezing. I remember my mother chasing me all over the house in the winter with these dorky knit caps and yelling, "Don't go outside without your cap! You lose fifty per cent of your body heat off the top of your head!" I would yank those stupid looking caps down on my head as I went out the door and yank them off my head as soon as I was out of my mother's sight. One day I mentioned what Mama said about losing body heat off the top of my head, to my father-in-law. Dr. Rivers, a pediatrician, said, "Your mother was right. The best way to keep your feet warm in the winter is to wear a cap."

Walker didn't like my cap. He said, "You look like your name should be Robespierre."

"Who is Robespierre?" I asked.

"I don't know. Some French dude with a stupid looking cap."

"Well, you don't have to like my cap. I'm wearing it because my head stays cold, and believe me, I look better with it than without it...."

Girlfriend advice: There are a few ways to make being bald a little easier. When you look straight on into your mirror, you only see a portion of the sides of your head. On the top you just see a few inches back. So, if being bald is getting you really depressed, then just don't look at your whole head bald. Stay away from three way mirrors that show the back of your head. You can wear a little soft knit cap to bed. Keep your wig on your bedside table. When you first wake up in the morning, sit up in bed , take off your sleeping cap and put on your wig before you get out of bed. When you get to the bath- room mirror, you can comb out your wig. This way you can go

through chemotherapy without seeing yourself bald.

Here is another suggestion, do not buy a human hair wig. Everyone I talked to that had used a human hair wig during chemo said it was a royal pain in the neck. They had to wash it, roll it and style it just as much as they did before on their real hair. A synthetic wig requires less washing and styling. You will love how much free time you have when you get a synthetic wig. And one more thing, buy a wig that has bangs long enough to cover up the area where your eyebrows are. Some girls draw on fake eyebrows, but I just felt more comfortable with long bangs. It's a whole lot easier. Think on the positive side, you have several months with no plucking eyebrows or shaving your legs!

A couple of days before Christmas, I started to have a sore throat. Then I developed a horrible hacking cough. I figured one of those germy people in the pharmacy line had given me some typical bug that was really laying me low because of the chemo. I spent most of my time bundled up on the couch in the front parlor by the Christmas tree. I couldn't take a chance on going out of the house because I was afraid of getting sicker than I was already. Then something good happened. My daughter, Laurel, became acquainted with a nice young man that loved to play the piano. Night after night Lewis would come over, and he and Laurel would play Christmas carols for me, while I sat on the couch all bundled up and wearing my "Ann Boleyn's about to get her head chopped off cap."

I looked forward to watching them sit on the piano stool, side by side, playing their little duets. I felt like I was living in a Jane Austin novel with all of my beautiful daughters and Lewis gracing my parlor. Sometimes Walker would sing while Laurel and Lewis played by the soft glowing warmth of the Christmas tree. I was really sick, but just being surrounded by lovely young faces made me feel that I was so very blessed.

A MIRACLE SAVED MY CHILD AND ME.

Dear Girlfriend,

So Christmas 2010 came. I was bald and had no breast on the left side, but I just put on Foxy and Marilyn and did my best to make a good Christmas for my little family. Again. We ate Kentucky Fried Chicken right out of the bucket on Christmas Eve while we watched "It' a Wonderful Life" and "Christmas in Connecticut" on television. On Christmas Morning, Walker hollered up the stairs, "Go back to bed! Santa Claus didn't come!" But of course he had. At Christmas dinner we ate turkey and the girls turned their noses up at the Waldorf salad. Then we had a scavenger hunt for money. My college aged daughters ran all over the downstairs, laughing and squealing like little girls as they tore the house apart looking for five dollars bills that I had hidden in the manger scene that was on the piano and on the Christmas tree.

New Year's Eve came and went with no celebration. No party. No anything. I was trying to stay away from people so I wouldn't catch the flu that was going around Macon. January was cold and gray and dreary. My third chemotherapy infusion was on January 10,2011. I sat in my recliner all wrapped up in a blanket, just looking around at all the sick people. The resilience of the human spirit amazed me. Here were all these people, fighting their own private battles, with their own bodies, but they never complained. Never did I ever hear anybody complaining in a doctor's waiting room or at the chemotherapy infusion center. If anything, I saw people come hobbling in looking like they could just give up the ghost any minute, but they would wave and say, "How's it going?" or "Good morning!" or "Is it cold enough for you out there?" And I would think,

"How do they do it? How do they just act like there is nothing wrong with them?"

I closed my eyes as I floated away on my Saint Happy Drug. I thought about all those people, in all those recliners, and I answered my own question in my head. I thought to myself, "These people have faith. These people have had something happen to them in their lives, that made them believe that God was going to take care of them. They might not be on this earth much longer, but they are not afraid." I was afraid. I was so so so afraid of death. I once again asked myself, "Why am I sitting out here on a big rock called Earth, just spinning around a big ball of fire, billions of miles from anything but more rocks and more balls of fire? What am I doing here?"

Of course everybody who has ever lived has asked this same question, and nobody really knows the exact answer to the question. The only thing I know to say is that we are here because God wants us to be here. This life is a gift. Then, I once again asked myself why did God allow me to suffer through having cancer? I have already come to the conclusion that if we could see the total picture we would understand, but I don't think God sat down and created cancer just to torture us. It could be that part of the answer is that God gave man freewill. It was up to us to be good stewards of the air and water and food supplies of this earth. Maybe we have not been such good stewards.

Maybe we have polluted our air and water and food supplies to the point that our bodies are just going crazy on a cellular level. Maybe we drink too much alcohol, take too much estrogen, and eat too much refined sugar etc. Maybe all this is not God's fault. Maybe cancer is rampant on Earth because of the choices we humans have made for thousands and thousands of years. Maybe we are not breathing what people are supposed to breathe. Maybe we are not eating what people are supposed to eat. Maybe we are not drinking what people are supposed to drink. And for these reasons our cells are not doing what our cells are supposed to do. Our cells are freaking out because of the environment that we have made for them. God didn't create a dirty planet. We did. God didn't create fruits and vegetables that have been sprayed with all sorts of pesticides. We did. So maybe I had no right to blame God for my cancer. Maybe people caused this epidemic, not God.

All I know is that there is a God, a loving God, who does watch over us. As I sat there in that recliner and I watched all those people who looked like they would be leaving this earth very soon, I listened to them talk. I heard them comforting each other. I saw strength like I had never witnessed before. I knew that they didn't just think God would take care of them. They knew it. I thought back over my life and racked my brain for a time that I was shown that God would take care of me. I tried to remember if I had ever experienced a miracle that proved to me that God would take care of me, and then I remembered the miracle. Then I knew that there was a God who would be there to take care of me, whether I survived my cancer or not.

This is the story of my miracle that I want to share with you. I do believe that everybody who has ever lived has experienced things that cannot be explained. Most people just write these experiences off as "coincidences." Most people don't want to admit that they have experienced something that cannot be explained because they don't want people to think they are lying or that they are just plain nuts. Well, I'm going to tell you something that happened to me and if you think I made this up, you are wrong. I promise this is the truth.

When I was in my twenties, I started trying to get pregnant. After a whole year of trying, I still was not pregnant. I decided to go to a fertility specialist. I went to a fertility specialist for six years. I wanted to have a baby more than anything else in the world, but no matter what the fertility specialists did, I just could not get pregnant. I had been on a fertility drug for quite a long time that was supposed to make me ovulate when I started seeing flashing lights and developed blind spots in my vision. My doctor told me that I was at the end of the road. He was afraid that if I kept on taking these drugs, I might have a stroke. So that was that.

I was devastated. I just could not get pregnant. So I prayed, "Okay, God. You know I did my best, but I can't have a baby. If you want me to have children, then you are going to have to take over because my heart has been broken every month for seven years! I can't do this anymore!" Then one day I was walking into the Macon Health Club with my friend Grace. Just as we were walking in the door, Grace's mother-in-law, Jeanne, was walking out the door. Now, let me stop here and say that if we had walked through that door one minute before, or one minute later, we would not have run into Jeanne and my entire life would have been different.

When we ran into Jeanne, my friend Grace said, "Jeanne, let me introduce you to my friend Suzan. Suzan wants a baby really bad, so if y'all ever get any babies that need to be adopted down at the church, let her know." You see, there was an adoption agency at Jeanne's church. We exchanged pleasantries and Jeanne was gone. The months rolled by and rolled by but still I had no little bundle in my empty arms.

Then one day I came in the door from work and Walker said, "I hesitate to tell you this because I can't bear to see you get hurt again...."

"Is it a baby? Walker, tell me! You have to tell me!" I begged.

"I don't know if we can get her...."

"Oh God! Tell me! Tell me!" I grabbed his arm and squeezed it so tight. "Please tell me!"

"Okay, but please, Suzan, please don't get excited, we might not be able to get her. Grace's mother-in-law told Grace that they have a baby girl at the church who is up for adoption. She said her mother-in-law saw the baby with the foster parents and immediately thought of you...."

"Oh Walker, it's our baby!!!" Before he could stop me I turned around and ran out the front door. I didn't even get in my car. I ran all the way to the Presbyterian church that was several blocks from our house. When I got there I just ran right in the door of their adoption agency and said as I tried to catch my breath from running, "You have my baby!!!"

The rest is history. I got the prize! After seven long years of trying to get pregnant, I put the whole problem in God's lap and before I could turn around, I had a beautiful baby girl. We named her Laurel Grace. Laurel means "victorious, strong and enduring", Grace means, " a gift from God." I was the happiest person on the entire planet. I was ecstatic! We adopted Laurel in August of 1988 when she was six weeks old. You see, as hard as I tried to get pregnant, I could not get pregnant. As soon as I stopped trying and said, "Lord, thy will be done," a baby came into my life. God wanted me to have children, but just not the way I thought it would happen.

Now I'm also going to tell you about the miracle that saved not only

Baby Laurel's life, but also my own. When Laurel was about eight months old, we had some extremely cold weather. Our house was old and we heated with floor furnaces. At night sometimes our house would get chilly. Since we were expecting really low temperatures that night, I put Laurel to bed and put a small child's sleeping bag over her. The bag was unzipped, so I thought it would be safe to use it as a heavy blanket. She went to sleep and I tiptoed out the door to my own bed. The next morning, before the sun came up, I was awakened by a sound. I lay in the bed with my eyes closed. I knew the sound, but I could not figure out why I was hearing it.

The sound was a music box that was inside of a porcelain doll that was on Laurel's mantlepiece. Now, if it had been playing some ghostly old song this could be a spooky story, but the song was ,"We've Only Just Begun" by the Carpenters. I was just, as I said, lying there in bed wondering how that music box had gotten turned on, when I was suddenly overpowered by a feeling inside me that said, "Hurry!!! Go check the baby!!!" I jumped out of bed and ran down the hall to her room as fast as I could. When I got to her bed, I saw that the sleeping bag was wrapped tightly around her head and body. All I could see were her two tiny little feet sticking out. I grabbed the sleeping bag and yanked it off as fast as I could. As soon as her head was out of the bag, she gasped for breath. She had been suffocating down in that sleeping bag. I grabbed her up into my arms and burst out crying. I fell to my knees as I cradled her and rocked her in my arms. All I could say was, "Thank you, God! Oh God! Thank you! Thank you! Thank you!!!"

I never gave the poor child a blanket for years. She slept in footie pajamas. Girlfriend, that music box was inside a doll that I had had for many years. To turn on the music box, I had to take the doll, turn her upside down and wind a key that was on the doll's back. In all the years that I had had the doll it had never started to play without me winding it up. Laurel is now twenty four years old, and that music box has never turned on one time again, unless I wound it up. Now you can say that was a coincidence, but I think it was a miracle.

I think that God knew that if I walked in and found my baby dead, suffocated in a blanket that I had put on her, I would have died along with her. God knew just how much I could stand and he saved my child and me because it was just not time for either one of us to go. Try to remember the miracle that happened in your life. Try to think of a time that something you could not explain protected you. Maybe at the time it happened you simply brushed it off as a coincidence, but if you really think about it, I'm sure you can think of a time that God has proven that He has you under his protection. When you look back on that time, when you reflect on it often, it will help you to overcome your fears. Fear. Fear of death, was my biggest obstacle to overcome while battling cancer. Thinking about how God woke me up and let me know to go check on Baby Laurel, and the prayers of my relatives and friends, lifted me up when I was afraid. I know now that I need not fear for God protects us all.

Girlfriend advice: Recognizing the miracles of protection that you have experienced in your life, and people praying for you, will get you through your fears. Prayer will get you through cancer.

This is a Facebook message that I posted on February1, 2011, the night before my last chemo infusion:

"Hey, everybody! Tomorrow at one o'clock I have my LAST chemo. I have done amazingly well with it so far and I think that is because of your prayers. So, please, once again, pray for me tomorrow. No matter what they do to my body, I manage to get through it. Please pray that this cancer will all be gone and I won't be afraid. I keep this scripture close, "Your troops will be with you on your day of battle."{Psalm 110}. Y'all are my troops! Love to all! Suzan."

I posted this message on Facebook the next day while I was doing my last chemo.

"Y'all saved me again. I woke up this morning unafraid. I am doing chemo now. I'm in a recliner all wrapped up in a warm blanket. I feel like a burrito! They just came by and put something in my IV bag to make me "feel good." I don't know what that stuff is, but wow! I feel good now! I keep singing this little song in my head to the tune of "You're in the Army Now". My version goes like this: "I'm in the chemo chair...I don't have any hair...Wearing my wig...Jiggity jig...I'm in the chemo chair!" When y'all were praying for me not to be afraid, you must have prayed me up some really good dope. What did they put in that bag? And it was legal too! Holy Moly! They should just put that stuff in the water system of the whole wide world. I feel like they have just announced that the IRS has been done away with and there will be no more income tax. Thanks again for praying me through chemo. "A friend loves at all times, and a brother is born for adversity." {Proverbs 17: 17} Your prayers for me at this time have made you all my brothers. Thank you from the pit of my soul."

I found out that the "feel good" drug was Ativan. If you get scared during chemo, ask your doctor about putting some Ativan in your IV bag. Whoa Nellie!!!

GIRL, ALWAYS PAY WITH CASH!

Dear Girlfriend,

My last chemo infusion was in February, 2011. Yippee! When I began doing chemo back in November, food tasted horrible. By March, food started to taste normal again I started eating everything that wasn't nailed down. Oh my gosh! Everything tasted so good! Well, everything had been tasting good to Walker for quite some time, and I must admit that I had been nagging him about eating too many sweets. Like I told you before, I host a Bible study group at my house every Friday. We do a lot of visiting at those meetings and we take turns bringing desserts. It just so happened that my sense of taste came back to me on a Friday when my friend Lisa brought a dessert called "Cherry Berries on a Cloud." Now, tell me, doesn't that sound like something mixed up by June Cleaver herself?

So, I must warn you. When your chemo is finally over, you just may have a strong craving for sweets, because sweets have tasted nasty for months. I ate two big helpings of "Cherry Berries on a Cloud" because it tasted so good. That just turned on my post chemo craving for sweets. After Bible, I was supposed to drive over to meet Walker at Fairy Ring Cottage. As I drove down the road, I just could not stop craving sugar. And, after going through chemo, didn't I just deserve a large chocolate malt with extra extra malt? So, I went to the drive through window at the Dairy Queen in Thomaston and got me a large chocolate malt with extra, extra malt and paid for it with my debit card. Then I tooled on down the road feeling like I had robbed a bank or something. I had to drive very slowly though so that I could finish the malt before I got to our property.

When I got to our property I didn't know what to do with the large paper cup because I didn't want Walker to see it. So, for the first time in my life, I chunked it out of the car window. It was on our land and I had every intention of going back to get it when he wasn't around. I figured I could burn it up in the fireplace. So, later on that evening Walker said, "Well, Boo Boo, I want to take you out for a nice big dinner since your food finally tastes good again. You should have a nice big juicy steak!"

I was just about to pop after two heaping helpings of "Cherry Berries on a Cloud" and my large chocolate malt with extra extra malt, but we got in his truck and headed out the gate of our property.

As we drove through the gate he said, "Would you look at that! Some jerk threw their Dairy Queen cup out there! I try so hard to keep this place clean and somebody is always throwing their trash out the window. That makes me so mad!" I just slunk down in my seat. I felt like I should confess, but I just muttered, "Oh, I'll pick it up later...."

Unfortunately for me, Walker does the checkbook stuff online. Boy is that Dairy Queen in Thomaston fast! I walked into the kitchen the next morning and he said as he pointed at his computer screen, "So it was YOU! YOU threw the Dairy Queen cup out your window! Here's the debit showing up on the computer! You're busted!" I hate computers. They won't let me get away with anything. I felt like Lucy with Ricky Ricardo saying, "Lucy! You got some splaining to do...." I told this story to my girlfriends one day at lunch and they all said, "Girl, haven't you learned yet... always pay with cash?!!!"

I AM A LIAR AND A THIEF.

Dear Girlfriend,

I made it through chemo and none of it was as bad as I thought it was going to be. I did get a bladder infection and I did get a bad case of bronchitis, but since I was religious about taking my Zofran, I experienced no nausea. Food tasted horrible, but that was just a bother, not a torment. I did get tired sometimes, but not too bad. My hair fell out, but with my cap and Foxy, being bald wasn't so awful. In short, the anticipation of chemo was worse than going through chemo. It just really and truly wasn't as bad as I thought it was going to be. I promise. If I can do it, so can you!

A few weeks passed and my hair started to come back. I must tell you that I felt like Harry the dirty dog. You see, when I'm not battling cancer, I'm a librarian in an elementary school. Although I have read plenty of Shakespeare, Curious George is more my speed. My all time favorite book is <u>Harry the Dirty Dog</u>. I have only stolen one thing in my entire life, if you don't count that tadpole that I took from our neighbor's pond when I was a little girl. Of course,that really doesn't count because as soon as he started to look droopy, I crawled back through Mrs. Scott's bushes and put him back in her pond. I worried all night that she was going to find "Taddy" belly up and call my mother to rat on me. She never called.

It was a different story with <u>Harry</u>. <u>Harry</u> was my all time favorite book when I was seven years old. Harry was a white dog with black spots. One day Harry went out on the town and got very dirty. It was sliding down the coal chute that really did it. You see, Harry changed from a white dog with black spots to a black dog with white spots. I thought that was the funniest thing I had ever heard. I remember sitting up in bed reading <u>Harry</u> over and over and laughing out loud. I was very easily entertained when I was seven and I wish my life were still so simple.

Since I was so in love with Harry, I checked him out of my school library three times in a row. On the third check out, the librarian told me that was the last time I could check Harry out. I was devastated. I was the youngest of six children and my mother didn't buy me presents except on Christmas and my birthday. If I had asked her to buy me a copy of Harry she probably would have, but I couldn't take a chance and blow my cover in case she refused. So, on the next Tuesday, library day, I hid Harry under my bed and trotted off to school.

When my class went to the library, I told the librarian a bald faced lie. "I lost Harry the Dirty Dog." She looked at me with suspicion, but told me to bring three dollars the next week to pay for the book. Whew! I was a thief. A liar and a thief. My conscience told me that I had done wrong, but I hit my mother up for the three dollars and kept my beloved Harry. After a few days I was even bold enough to read my beloved Harry right out in the living room. How could my mother, with a house full of children, ever notice the title of the book I was reading? I'm sure that she was just thrilled that I was happy to just sit and read and not out sliding down a coal chute like Harry.

So why did I feel like Harry when my hair finally started to come back? When I lost all my hair from the chemo my hair was brown. Well, it was mostly brown. I admit that I colored it, but it was mostly brown. When my hair came back from chemo it was mostly white. I felt just like Harry. I had changed from a brown dog with white spots to a white dog with brown spots. Maybe this was pay back for being a liar and a thief. It had finally caught up with me.

Walker loved my new hair, which was only about a quarter of an inch long. Every time I'd walk by him he would grab me and rub my head. "You are so cute! Your head feels just like a puppy belly!"

I growled at him. Puppy belly was not exactly the look I was aiming for. When my hair fell out only half way down, Laurel said that I looked like Ben Franklin. Now I was being called a puppy belly. You never know where life is going to take you. My hair continued to grow until it was extremely thick and extremely curly. It came back so much better than it was before I did chemo. I do color it brown, but it is just so soft that Walker can't keep his hands out of it. Getting to this point was a little dramatic, but it was worth it... I know you can make it, just don't give up!

SEX? YOU'VE GOT TO BE KIDDING!!!

Dear Girlfriend,

My last chemo was February 3, 2011.When I had my first MRI after I was diagnosed with cancer, the test detected masses in both my bladder and my kidneys.   I then went to a urologist that did an ultrasound and determined that I had polyps in my bladder and cysts in my kidneys. He said they were quite common and nothing to worry about. I mentioned this to my oncologist after I had chemo and he said, "After age fifty, cysts in the kidneys are very common. The only way to find out if those polyps in your bladder are benign is to have them taken out."

So for my peace of mind, I had those polyps in my bladder removed in April, 2011.   They were benign.   That was surgery number ten.   My urologist told me that to have a healthy urinary tract, I should drink cranberry juice or take cranberry capsules daily.   Since I started taking cranberry capsules every day, I have had no more urinary tract infections. I highly recommend cranberry capsules to everybody I know. I made sure that the capsules contained no soy protein.   All the vitamins and supplements I take have no soy protein because soy protein contains estrogen. Soy oil, which is in just about everything you buy, is supposedly okay, but it's the soy protein that you might want to avoid. Talk to your dietician about soy. I avoid estrogen like the plague.

The next month, May 2011, I went back to my oncologist, Dr. Pippas, " Your cancer is estrogen driven. I really think you need to have your ovaries removed and change over to Arimidex to block any estrogen in your body." My first thought was that I might just go ahead and have a complete hysterectomy. I went back to my gynecologist, Teri, and told her my idea.

"You don't want to have your uterus removed. If I take out your uterus, you could have problems with bladder control. Don't worry. Breast cancer doesn't go to your uterus."

So surgery number eleven was scheduled to remove my ovaries. This surgery was a piece of cake. If your doctors want you to have your ovaries removed, don't be afraid. My surgery was done laproscopically and I had no pain at all. I was up and around the very next day. The problem with having my ovaries removed was the vaginal dryness that followed. This was no small problem. I was afraid that if I had my ovaries removed, I would have no more sex drive. I was afraid that I would feel like a spayed cat laid out in the sunshine... and actually that might have been easier. If I could manage to get past only having one breast and having puppy belly hair, then my next obstacle to having sex was to overcome that awful vaginal dryness. When I say dry I mean the Sahara Desert had nothing on me. Any attempt to have sex was so excruciating that we just gave up.

"Sex is absolutely impossible, we have tried every lubricating product in the drugstore," I lamented to one of my girlfriends. "Have you tried olive oil?" she asked. "Olive oil? How in the world am I supposed to get olive oil up there?" "With a turkey baster?" I just looked at her and we both laughed. "I'll have to think of something else."

Walker said, "What about WD-40? That always works on rusty hinges." Now, you see why you should go to your girlfriend for advice. "I know you're getting desperate, Walker, but I better not try the WD-40." "Oh, well, it was just a thought..." he said. After trying every single product at the pharmacy that did not contain estrogen I was out of ideas.

Walker and I mentioned the problem to Dr. Pippas. I was totally embarrassed and humiliated, but was desperate enough to ask him if we could use Ora-jel internally to numb the pain. "Ora-jel would be safe to use for pain. Vitamin E oil or olive oil would be safe to use for lubrication. Don't give up. Keep on trying," That was easy to say but difficult to do. Every "try" ended in tears. It was absolutely horrible. I think painful intercourse was probably one of the worst parts of the whole breast cancer battle. If you are having this problem, all I know to say is slow and steady wins the race. Don't give up that special part of your life. Just keep on trying until you can manage having sex. Don't let cancer strip that away from you too. Taking little out-of-town trips, just the two of you, really will give you a chance to relax and enjoy being alone together.

You can ask your doctor about Vitamin E vaginal suppositories. They work better than anything else I could find for vaginal dryness. You can order them through your pharmacist or online. Vitamin E oil is also very helpful. It's one hundred per cent all natural and contains no extra ingredients that could irritate your skin.

Another problem I experienced after having my ovaries removed was my skin tone. To be fifty-four, I was still pretty firm. After my ovaries were removed, I noticed that I started to feel soft. My muscle tone just started to go and I felt like a deflated balloon. I couldn't exercise as strenuously as I needed to until all of my surgeries were far behind me.

Girlfriend advice: If you have your ovaries removed and you can't have sex due to the pain and your body feels like Jell-o, don't jump off a bridge. Keep saying those magic words, "This is only temporary". Talk to your doctor about painful intercourse. Start exercising as soon as you possibly can after surgery to firm up your muscles.

They don't call having cancer a "battle" for nothing! Breast cancer will try to take everything from you. Your inner peace. Your beauty. Your sexuality. Your personality. Your life. Don't let cancer win! You have to keep on fighting. Don't give up! Try praying to the Holy Spirit. The Holy Spirit will give you strength and peace of mind so that you won't just throw in the towel . Ask for peace and it will be given to you. When you first wake up in the morning, pray this simple prayer for yourself, "No pain. No fear. No death." Pray this simple prayer all day every day whenever you are feeling down. Also, try praying this simple prayer daily: "Holy Spirit dwell in me." One day you will wake up, and much to your surprise you will feel better.

AN OLD SOUTHERN TRADITION: A COOL WET RAG.

Dear Girlfriend,

By the middle of June 2011, my hair was about an inch long. Now, I must remind you that I never told my mother I had cancer. The only thing I could think of that would be worse than having cancer, would be one of my daughters having cancer. I knew that my mother would suffer immeasurably if she watched me battle cancer, so I just put the word out on the family gossip line that everybody should hide my cancer from Mama. I have a huge family. I have five brothers and sisters. All of my siblings have children and now all of those children are having families. When we all get together, there are about seventy of us. On June 14, 2011, my mother, Mary Pacetty Lampp, turned ninety years old. I decided to host a birthday party at Fairy Ring Cottage and invite all the relatives. I invited my mother's sisters' children as well as all of our branch of the family.

On the day of the party the thermostat read ninety- five degrees. My wig, Foxy, is made of some sort of synthetic material. It was so hot I could barely stand to wear it. All inside and outside of the cottage, sixty-two of my close relatives were arriving from all over the country. I've never seen so many babies at one place in my life! We were all talking and hugging and laughing while we waited for one of my nieces to arrive from Columbus with Mama. Walker hollered, "Hey, everybody! They'll be here in a minute! Let's line both sides of the driveway!" So all sixty-two of us headed outside in that ninety-five degree heat to greet the birthday girl when she arrived.

After about ten minutes of standing out in that sticky sweltering heat, I started having hot flashes. Oh joy. I had been taking Arimidex, the estrogen blocker, and every time I got hot I would start feeling like fire ants were biting me from head to toe. So there I was trying to pull off this party while feeling like I was covered with stinging insects. I ran back in the house to the bathroom and yanked Foxy off of my head. I was drenched in sweat. I just stood at the sink and splashed cold water on my face and I knew that I just could not make it through the day wearing that wig. So I hid Foxy in the cabinet and ran back outside to join the relatives.

I had already given them some party horns, so when the car approached, they blew their horns and started clapping and shouting, "Happy Birthday!" to Mama. The car pulled up right in front of the cottage door and all of my mother's children, grandchildren and great grandchildren crushed around the car to greet her. She was laughing and hugging everybody. As I made my way through the crowd to hug her, she saw me. She just got this blank look on her face and said, "What in the world happened to your hair?"

Everybody just held their breathe as I replied, "I got a haircut and the lady got a little carried away...." Mama just looked bumfuzzled and said, "You're telling me. You need a wig!" The whole crowd just started laughing. My sister whispered in my ear, "If she only knew..."

> **Girlfriend advice: If you take an estrogen inhibitor, you might itch and feel like bugs are biting you when you get hot. This can be so discouraging. A friend of mine told me that her itchy feelings stopped after about a year, so don't despair. Always, even in the winter, wear sleeveless clothes with a sweater that you can take off easily. That way, if you have a hot flash or the bugs start biting, you can cool off. In the summer try to stay out of the heat as much as possible. If you exercise, do it inside in air-conditioning. Take cool baths. Hot showers will set you on fire. Never underestimate the power of an old southern tradition, a cool wet rag!**

By the first week of July, it had been thirteen months since my breasts had been removed. In those thirteen months I had been through the bilateral mastectomy, the staph infection, the left implant ripping out, the left implant being removed, my chest not healing for five months, chemo, going bald, bladder surgery, ovaries removed, hot flashes with bugs biting and painful intercourse. Whew! Now I faced the latissimus flap surgery, taking the tissue and skin from my back to help construct a new left breast. I felt like a horse that was just about to collapse right at the finish line....

LATISSIMUS DORSI MUSCLE FLAP SURGERY

Dear Girlfriend,

If radiation makes your skin so weak that it will probably not hold an implant, you may need to have a latissimus dorsi muscle flap surgery. That means that your surgeon will take a portion of the latissimus dorsi muscle from your back to help reconstruct a breast for you. The way he will do this is to move the muscle from your back, with the skin and the artery still attached, to your chest area. He basically will just push the muscle around you, under the skin on your side, from your back, to your chest area. An implant will be used under the muscle to finish making the breast.

I had this surgery in July 2011. This was surgery number twelve. Walker and I left Fairy Ring Cottage at 3:30 AM because we were told to arrive at the hospital at 4:30 AM. "I hate driving down to Columbus in the middle of the night. I just don't like arriving at the hospital in the pitch black dark," I told Walker as he drove me down Pine Mountain towards Columbus. "Everything just seems so much better to me if the sun is shining," I said. "Well, at least Dr. Naman won't be tired since you'll be his first surgery today."

We arrived at the hospital as instructed at 4:30AM. When we got to the waiting area where we were told to go, there was not one soul in sight. I just scrunched up in my chair and tried to talk myself out of making a run for it. I was tired of surgeries, but I wanted my new breast so badly that I talked myself into going through yet another major surgery. I was just about to fall asleep in my chair when I remembered something. "Oh! I almost forgot!" I said as I pulled a postcard out of my pocketbook.

All through my breast cancer treatment, I kept a postcard stuck to my refrigerator with a photograph of the statue *The David* on it. You see, David had become my hero. David slew Goliath. I figured if David could slay Goliath with the help of God, then I could slay cancer with the help of God. I sure could not slay cancer without God's help. "What are you doing with that postcard?" Walker asked. On the front of the postcard was the face of David looking up into the face of Goliath. On the back of the card was printed, Michelangelo's masterpiece: *The David*. Under that I had written, "Dear Dr. Naman, I want to be YOUR masterpiece, *The Suzan*. Walker just read the card and laughed.

About that time they called me back to put on the lovely gown and cap. I had become familiar with the whole routine. "Honey, just put these on and get up on that gurney," the nurse told me. Everybody was moving really fast that morning and before I knew what was happening, the IV was dripping into my port with some sort of happy drug. "Kiss her goodbye!" the nurse said. Walker kissed me on top of my head and they rolled me right on into the operating room. "Scoot yourself over onto the operating table," the nurse instructed. Right before they put me to sleep, I handed Dr. Naman the postcard. "Read this before you start," I said. The last thing I remember was him smiling at me.

When I woke up, I was in the recovery room. I remember complaining that my arm hurt a little but it wasn't too painful. I had been totally amazed at how little pain I had had through all my surgeries. The male nurse rolled me back to my room and I remember him telling Walker that I had asked him what kind of restaurant I was in. They were laughing about that as I was tucked into bed and given a morphine pump. In a little while Dr. Naman came in. I must have been dozing because when I opened my eyes, he was leaning over me saying, "How do you feel, 'The Suzan'?" I just smiled and dozed back off....

The next thing I remember was itching. I was itching like crazy all around my surgery site. The nurses came in and tried to console me, but I was having some sort of allergic reaction. I was so miserable I wanted to just tear that bandage off my chest and claw my skin off. I used the morphine pump, not because I was in pain, but because I thought it would help stop the itching. If only I had known then what I know now. It was the morphine that was making me itch. Morphine is an opiate and I had developed an allergic reaction to opiates. I had had itching with a couple of other surgeries, but nothing like this. To this day I can barely stand to think about how miserable I was. The sweet nurses put every kind of lotion they could think of around the top of the bandage, but nothing helped.

On the third day after surgery, Dr. Naman came to my room. "When can I go home?" I asked. "You can leave as soon as you give up the morphine pump," he answered. "Well, take it away. I haven't really had any pain, just this horrible itching that's about to drive me crazy!"

I left the hospital the next morning and Walker and I drove straight to a drugstore to get some Benadryl. Girlfriend, by the time we got back to Macon I was itching so bad I was in tears. "Walker, I can't stand this itching! I'm about to lose it! We've got to do something!" I was clawing my skin all around where those drains were coming out of my skin. Soon I noticed that blood was running down my side from where I had clawed my skin off.

When we got home I went right to the phone and made an appointment for the next day with a dermatologist. The night before that appointment was just about the most miserable night of my life. The drains that were attached to the plastic bulbs to collect the fluid from my reconstructed breast were very long, down past my knees. That night I climbed up the heavy wooden bedside step stool into our high antique bed. I couldn't sleep because I was itching so badly. After a while I got up to go to the bathroom with my long drains dragging along behind me. I wasn't wearing my little camisole that had the pockets in it for the drains because wearing the camisole interfered with my ability to scratch.

So as I was climbing back up that heavy step stool to get up onto the bed, my drains went down between the rungs of the stool. Don't ask me exactly what happened, but I somehow managed to flip that heavy stool up in the air as I went crashing down on the floor flat on my back. The step stool came crashing down between my legs and landed right on my pelvis. I screamed bloody murder and Walker jumped up to find me flat on my back with that big heavy stool between my legs tangled up with drains and bulbs every which way. I was crying and he was trying to untangle the mess I had made. "Boo Boo, what in the world have you done?" "I don't know what happened....that step stool just attacked me! I think I broke my hoo-ha!!!" I cried as Walker got me all untangled and helped me back into the bed.

The next morning I was black and blue all down my inner thighs and pelvis. I was able to get up and hobble around so I figured nothing was broken. Nothing was going to keep me from going to that dermatologist. I was practically out of my mind with itching. When we finally got in to see the dermatologist he could tell that I was really suffering by the skin that I had clawed off my side. He said, "You're having a major allergic reaction to something. Do you think it could be the surgical prep?"

"I don't have a clue. But if I don't stop itching soon, I'm really going to lose my mind!" I said as I clawed at my skin. Then the dermatologist took a tongue depressor and said, "I'm going to 'write' some letters on your back with this wooden tongue depressor. Let's just wait a minute and see what happens." Then he just took the tongue depressor and 'drew' letters across my back. In a minute he said to Walker, "Look at this!" I could hear Walker say "Wow! Every letter is raised up in big red welts." The doctor said, "That's called dermographia. She is really having a major reaction. I want her to take a combination of Zantac and Allegra."

"Isn't Zantac for heartburn?"

"Yes. But it's also an antihistamine. Zantac and Allegra are two different types of antihistamines. Combined, they just might stop the itching. I also want you to get some of this ointment, Clobetasol Propionate USP, 0.05%. Together maybe you'll get some relief."

"Man, I hope so!" I said as I continued to claw at my skin while big red welts appeared everywhere I scratched. On the way home we got my prescriptions. When we got back to the house, I took off my clothes, put on the softest nightgown I could find and started to climb up on that step stool to get in bed. "Okay, you smart aleck stool! You sit right there and don't go jumping around!!!" Walker brought me the Zantac and Allegra and the ointment. "Who were you talking to?" he asked. "I was talking to that stool that tried to murder me," I said. "Oh. Well, it's just hard to find a good dependable stool these days," he said. "You're telling me." Walker gave me the pills and I took them. Then he helped me slather the ointment all around the bandage on my breast.

At that point I was not taking anything for pain and after a few days the itching stopped. I knew the Zantac and Allegra and the ointment were calming down my skin, but I just did not make the connection that the morphine and opiate based painkillers were what had caused it. If I had only known then what I know now....

In a few days I was back to see Dr. Naman to remove the bandage and get a look at my new breast. "Well, let's take a look," he said as he took off all the bandages. He handed me a mirror and I looked. " It's a lot higher than the other one," I said. "It will settle down into position over the next few months," Dr. Naman said. Girlfriend, considering what he had to work with, which was absolutely nothing, it was amazing. The old radiated skin had been removed. Going straight across my breast was an incision that was shaped like a football. That was the fresh skin that had been taken from my back. The muscle and the artery were still attached to this skin, but it really didn't have much feeling at that point. The scar on my back was a thin line about ten inches long. It had an area that was pooched out looking. Dr. Naman had called that area a "dog ear" and said that it could be fixed.

So the months of July and August rolled on by as my skin grew strong in it's new location. The incisions healed slowly, but they did heal.

Girlfriend advice: Since I had had so much trouble with my radiated skin not healing, I was afraid to put anything on the new incisions, like petroleum jelly to keep them soft. That was a bad mistake!!!With the latissimus flap surgery I was dealing with the skin that had been taken from my back. It was good strong skin, not radiated skin, so I should have kept the skin moist. Certain areas of the incision formed very hard thick scabs that made scars. So, if you have to have latissimus flap surgery, keep your incisions moist with Vaseline or Aquaphor to prevent scarring.

I SAW THE LIGHT!

Dear Girlfriend,

Everything seemed to be going along well when my ninety-year-old mother got sick. It started out as a simple bladder infection but she ended up in the hospital in acute renal failure. After a few days in the hospital, her doctors sent her back to the assisted living home. There was nothing else they could do. Everybody in the family came from all over the country to see her. She was not in a coma, but she was extremely hard to wake up. I moved into Fairy Ring Cottage once more so that I could be at my mother's side every day. My brothers and sisters and I were sure that Mama was dying. But, every time we could get her to wake up, we would give her just a swallow of Coca-Cola and a spoon of Campbell's cream of chicken soup.

Then one day after weeks and weeks of being only semi-conscious, she just completely woke up and said, "I need to get my hair fixed." My sister, Cea, wheeled her down the hall of the assisted living home to the beauty parlor to get her hair fixed. My friend Molly said, "Don't get excited. She probably just wants to look good laid out in her coffin." I figured Molly must be right and I relayed this message onto the family gossip tree. Everybody agreed that Molly's prognosis must be right. The beautician refused to let us pay her for the wash and set since it was her last time. Then Mama said, "I want some chocolate covered cherries." Cea gave her chocolate covered cherries and called to give me the good news that Mama had eaten something solid. "It's probably her last dying wish. She's always loved chocolate covered cherries," I told Walker. He nodded in agreement.

Hospice came. Father Patterson came to give her the last rites. I was beside myself with grief. I prayed and prayed that God would not let her be in any pain or fear and if it was her time to go, that he would take her to heaven to be with her mama and daddy and sisters who had gone on before her so many years ago. Then as the days dragged on and on and on, Mama woke up and said, "I've been out all night with Little Joe. His hair is completely white now...." Then she drifted back to sleep. When the Hospice nurse came I took her aside and said, "She's talking out of her mind. She thinks she was with Little Joe Cartwright from "Bonanza" last night." The nurse smiled and said, "What makes you think she wasn't?"

Then Mama wanted to watch TV. She seemed to know exactly what was going on with every show. The weeks just rolled by and Mama was still alive. Nobody could believe it. Her doctors thought for sure that she would die because her kidneys had almost completely stopped working, but somehow just giving her little sips of Coke got her kidneys cranked up again. There must be something good in Coca-Cola! It was totally amazing how she was just so close to death, but made a come back. So you really need to hang on to that old saying, "Where there's life there's hope."

Then on November 8, 2011, I had to get my chemotherapy port flushed. You see if you have a chemo port you must have it flushed with saline solution every month. Even though I was finished with chemotherapy my oncologist wanted me to keep the port in for a year post chemo just in case the cancer came back again. Having my port flushed every month had become very routine, but on that particular day something went wrong. Dr. Pippas said that he needed three vials of blood drawn. We went to a lab. When we got there my nurse was in a hurry. I don't know why she was doing everything so fast, but she said, "Just sit down right here. You're going to have to take off those pearls so I can get to your port." I took off my long strand of pearls and handed them to Walker. He was standing across the room wearing his forestry clothes, blue jeans, big heavy hiking boots and a plaid flannel shirt. He simply took the pearls and put them around his neck. They really didn't go with his outfit.

The nurse cleaned the area of my chest where my port was and then stuck a syringe full of saline solution into my port. Then she pushed the plunger in as fast as possible and drew back on the plunger as fast as possible. "I didn't get any blood," she said as she took off that syringe and inserted another one. Then she repeated the same procedure pushing in the saline and drawing out to get the blood super fast. Again she said, "I still didn't get any blood." At that point I said, "I'm feeling a very cold sensation in my neck." She said, "Oh, don't worry about that. Let me try again." So in very rapid fire succession she pushed in saline, pulled out blood, pushed in saline, pulled out blood, pushed in saline, pulled out blood. At that point I had five vials of saline trying to pump through my heart. All I remember saying was, "I'm going...."

Walker said that my eyes rolled back in my head, my cheeks became flaccid and started to quiver, my legs started to twitch, and I was out. Way way out. He caught me as I slumped forward and the nurse called for help. Then, according to Walker, the entire room was full of people, including six EMTs who had come in an ambulance. They were unable to get a pulse on me and proceeded to shoot atropine straight into my port to get my heart to start beating normally. I was out so cold that I was totally unaware that I had been picked up and lain on an examination table. I was somewhere else.

While Walker said that literally twenty people ran into the lab to work on bringing me back around, I remained completely unaware of what was going on with my body. All I remember was being completely surrounded by a warm, glowing light. I was totally peaceful, totally unafraid. What I was experiencing was so totally different than when I had been put to sleep for surgery all those many times. If you have ever been put to sleep,under general anesthesia, you know that while you are out, you experience nothing. You are completely, totally, unaware of everything that is happening. You don't remember thinking or feeling.

Whenever I wake up after surgery, I always ask, "When are you going to start?" Invariably, there is always a nice recovery room nurse who says, "Honey, it's all over." But this time was nothing like being put to sleep. My mind was wide awake and thinking and I could see. My body was laid out on a table with my eyes closed, but I was seeing bright, warm, glowing light and my mind was asking, "What is all this light?"

That's all I remember about being out. The next thing I remember was opening my eyes and hearing somebody say, "Her pulse is up to thirty-six!" There was an EMT over me saying, "Tell me your name! Tell me where you are!" I just lay there in complete peace and said, "I'm Suzan Rivers. Where is Walker?" Then I called out for Walker and he appeared and held my hand. The EMTs were trying to sit me up and put me on a stretcher to take me to the hospital. I said, "I can step down." So I sat up on the examination table as a group of people held on to me and helped me off the table and down onto the stretcher. Then as they started to wheel me away out the front of the building, I asked, "What happened?" They put me in the back of an ambulance and one of the EMTs jumped up into the ambulance with me. He closed the doors and we were off to the trauma ward of the hospital.

I just lay there in the ambulance as the EMT fired question after question at me, "Where do you live? What's your husband's name? How old are you? What day is it?" I answered all the questions and then I asked him, "What happened?" He just said, "You had an episode...." Then I remembered exactly what I had experienced being surrounded by that warm, glowing, peaceful light and I just asked him outright, "Did I die?" He just looked at me sort of funny and said, "Yes, ma'am. I think you did, but don't worry, you're going to be just fine. You're talking like you're fine."

We got to the hospital and they took me into the trauma area. There was a nice doctor who came and said, "We're going to run some tests to see if we can figure out what happened to your heart. What do you remember happening?" I told him that after the fifth syringe of saline was put into my port and three vials of blood were drawn out in very rapid succession, I told the nurse I was passing out. After that I didn't know what happened, I was somewhere else.

I stayed on the gurney the entire afternoon while they did a battery of tests. At the end of the afternoon, the doctor came back in and said, "Your heart is fine. I think you just had too much saline solution in your heart. That saline pretty much shut your heart down. You must have had some little bit of circulation going on though, because the atropine got it back up and going. If it had completely stopped they would have had to use other means to get you going." We thanked him and left.

When we got back up to Fairy Ring Cottage, I noticed that I was still feeling extremely calm. I was actually happy. It had been so long since I had felt truly happy that I had forgotten what it felt like. I went to bed that night feeling like there was a nice warm, pleasant glow all around me. As I snuggled up to Walker I said, "Oh, where is my pearl necklace? I remember giving it to you and you put it on...."

"Yeah, there I was with my jeans, my boots and my flannel shirt wearing your lovely strand of pearls. Then twenty people came pouring into the lab when I realized I was still wearing the pearls."

"Well, were you embarrassed?"

"Are you kidding? I was too scared to be embarrassed, but I did take them off and slip them into my pocket as fast as I could once I noticed I still had them on!" We had a good laugh about that and went on to sleep.

The next morning when I woke up, I still felt totally at peace. I wasn't just happy, I was downright euphoric. "I haven't ever felt so good. I want to dance!" I told Walker as I put a dance CD in the player. Then I just started dancing. I danced all around the cottage and right out the front door, which is out in the middle of the woods where no neighbors could see me and say, "Why is that crazy woman dancing around in her nightgown?"

"Walker! I feel so good! I've never felt so happy! I'm not scared anymore!!! I'm just not scared anymore!!!" It was wonderful. I must have swallowed some of the light. I've never felt so utterly happy and peaceful before in my life. Walker just watched me dance all over the house and then he danced some with me. He hugged me and kissed me and said, "It's so good to see you happy and not suffering."

I called my sister, Cea, and told her everything that had happened.

"Did you see God?"

"No."

"Did you see angels?"

"No."

"Did you see any of your friends who have died, or Daddy, or any saints or anybody at all?"

"No. I just saw light. Warm, glowing, peaceful light. I was so peaceful. I still feel it. I just don't feel afraid of dying anymore. Passing away was so peaceful."

"I had a friend once who had a near death experience and all he saw was bright, warm light. He thought it was the fires of hell," she laughed.

"Well, if there is a hell, this was not it. Cea, I felt so good that my first thought when I became conscious was ,'Why did they have to wake me up?'" I said.

"Wow. How do you feel now?"

"I feel like I hope I never stop feeling like I do right now. I feel indescribably wonderful."

"Oh, Suzan, I hope it lasts." But it did not. I felt the greatest peace I had ever known that day, but when I got up the next morning it was gone. All gone. I was back to normal. Bummer. I told Walker that the euphoric feeling was all gone. He said, "Boo Boo, maybe God gave you a gift. Maybe he gave you just the slightest glimmer of what happens when you go to heaven. Maybe he wants you to stop grieving over your mama and to stop being afraid of your own death." "You might be right," I said. I just wish I had seen somebody that I knew while I was out, but I didn't. I wish that I had seen Daddy, or one of my girlfriends or an angel or Jesus, just somebody, but all I saw was light." "Well, that's more than most people ever experience," he said.

I have often thought about the day Jesus was crucified. The apostles went and hid because they were so terrified that they would be taken into custody and also crucified. Can you just imagine how scared they were? But then Jesus appeared to them. They were able to touch Him and feel the wounds in His hands and His side. After that they didn't have to operate on faith anymore. They didn't just "believe" that life is eternal, they absolutely knew that they would live forever. There is a big difference between thinking that life is eternal and having seen absolute proof. I have never seen Jesus in flesh and blood. I, after my cancer diagnosis, was terrified of death because I had never seen a person who had died and then come back in the flesh like Jesus did when he appeared to the apostles. You and I have to operate on faith, but the apostles operated for the rest of their lives, not on faith, but on absolute proof.

They had seen the risen Christ. They touched Him. They talked with Him. They even ate with Him. After that they had no fear of death. They went forth and preached the good news about Jesus and literally allowed themselves to be caught and tortured and martyred. Why would they allow this to happen? They could have laid low and shut up and not been arrested by the authorities, or overtaken by angry mobs, but that is not what they did. The reason they stood up and taught about Christ was that by letting the apostles see Him in the flesh, alive and well after He had been in the grave, Jesus took away the apostles fear of death.

I can't sit here and tell you that I have no fear of death. That would be a lie. But, I can tell you that whatever that was that I experienced, while my heart had all but stopped beating, was the most wonderful peace I have ever known. I felt no fear, no pain and no death. I was thinking and seeing even though my eyes were closed. I hope this gives you some peace of mind. I experienced no break in seeing or feeling. If anything, my seeing and feeling were intensified. All along, my mantra since I was diagnosed with cancer has been, "No pain. No fear. No death." And that is exactly what I experienced.

SOMETHING HAS GONE BAD WRONG IN HOLLYWOOD!

Dear Girlfriend,

On Thanksgiving Day, 2011, my sister Cathy stayed with Mama while I had all of Walker's side of the family come to Fairy Ring Cottage. Just remember, having cancer gives you no time out. There were about thirty of us. Thanksgiving in the woods is great because you can sit out on our huge back porch and actually see deer and turkey pass by. The day after Thanksgiving we put a tiny little tree in the cottage and then went back to Macon to decorate. Christmas 2011 was my fourth Christmas since I had been diagnosed with cancer and I was still not finished with my reconstruction.

I was determined to make Christmas just as memorable as always. We put "the giants", Mary, Joseph, Baby Jesus and all the rest of the huge figurines on the piano. Again. We decorated a ten foot tall Christmas tree in the parlor. Again. Laurel's friend Lewis, who had been around every night during Christmas time the year before, was now Laurel's boyfriend, not just a friend. A lot of changes can take place in a year. Mama was still alive and had her right mind, but she was bedridden.

I took her a little Christmas tree and decorated her room at the assisted living home. Day after day I would sit and watch episode after episode of "Bonanza" and "Mash." Every commercial on her Channel 54 advertised things for elderly people. We would sit and watch advertisements for scooter chairs, grabbers, alert systems, walk-in bathtubs and the like. I thought that Mama really enjoyed this channel with all her old favorite shows. Then one day when we were on our third episode of "Three's

Company," a commercial came on for snap-on teeth. The elderly man on TV would take these fake teeth and just push them on over his old teeth. Mama was watching intently and I thought she was really interested in those snap on teeth when she turned to me with a serious expression on her face and said, "Something has gone bad wrong in Hollywood."

Christmas Eve came. We went to mass. Again. We came back home and ate Kentucky Fried Chicken right out of the bucket while we snuggled up in the TV room watching *Christmas in Connecticut*. Again. We all know every line by heart and Laurel and I say our favorite lines in unison. So we're the little dork family, but who cares? At least we're all together. When we watch *It's a Wonderful Life* Laurel always says, "I'm like George Bailey. I want to get out of here and go see the world!" I always say, "Yeah, you'll be the one to end up spending your whole life right here in little old Macon, Georgia!" "No way!" she says every year.

On Christmas morning, my fourth Christmas morning since my diagnosis, the girls and I sat on the top step of the staircase and waited for Walker to holler up, "Go back to bed! Santa Claus didn't come!" And of course he was lying. We gathered around the Christmas tree, still in our pajamas with our hair standing out all which- a- way. I was assigned to sit on the floor and hand out the presents. Walker said, "Open that little box." It was a cross necklace. "I thought you could use a little added protection," he said. "I can use all the protection I can get!" I replied. Lewis, Laurel's boyfriend, was the new face at the Christmas table. He actually ate some Waldorf Salad. Nobody else touched the stuff. I threw the rest away...Again. Thank God for again!!!

Girlfriend advice: Don't let your fear of cancer killing you ruin your life. Keep up your traditions just like you did before you had cancer. And on a medical note, make sure that whoever does your port flushes goes slowly and carefully. A heart is not supposed to run on saline solution.

CHEMOTHERAPY PORT REMOVED. YIPPEE!!!

Dear Girlfriend,

Just three days after Christmas, December 28, 2011, I went to a surgery center to have yet another surgery. Number thirteen. This surgery was to remove the saline implant that was on my right side and replace it with a silicone implant. You see, if a woman has breast implants to make her breasts larger, then the implant is placed under her real tissue. That means that the breast will still feel very natural after the implant is in place, because it is covered with real tissue. When you have had a mastectomy, your real tissue has been removed, so all you are left with is your breast skin, the implant, and a thin material that your surgeon will place over the implant. So, what happened in my case was that the saline implant that Dr. Naman put in when my breast tissue was removed did not cooperate. Dr. Naman had done everything just right, but the saline implant felt like a bag of water. The only thing missing was the goldfish. Glub... Glub....

My breast felt like a bag of water because that is basically what it was. Without any breast tissue to cover that saline implant, it felt like a bag of water, and it acted like a bag of water. If I were standing up, it looked fine, but if I lay down, it would basically walk over to the side of my chest and jump off into my armpit! It also had very deep creases because it was behaving like a bag of water.

Now, there are two different types of implants. I had opted for the saline on the first surgery, but since it would not behave like a breast, probably because my skin was so very thin, Dr. Naman said we could remove the saline implant and replace it with a silicone implant. That surgery, as I said, was on December 28, 2011. That surgery was the most miserable of all my surgeries, not from pain, but from itching. My allergy to opiates had been getting a little worse with each surgery, but by this one it was full blown.

From the minute I woke up from surgery I was itching so badly that I was about to lose it. Walker took me straight from the surgery center to Fairy Ring Cottage. I was again taking hydrocodone, an opiate based pain killer. For three days I suffered so much that all I could do was claw at my skin and cry. I went back to Dr. Naman to show him that I was again experiencing dermographia. If I "wrote" on my skin with my fingernail, you could read what I "wrote" as red welts appeared instantly. "I can tell you're really suffering," he said. "Maybe you are allergic to the pain meds. Try not to use the hydrocodone, just use Tylenol and see if it gets better."

So that is what I did. On New Year's Eve, Walker and I were alone at Fairy Ring Cottage while I cried all night from the sheer misery of itching. I thought back to the last New Year's Eve party we had given on December 31, 2007. So much had happened. Lumpectomy. Radiation that ruined my skin so that it would not heal. Both breasts removed. Both breasts reconstructed. Staph infection that could have killed me. Implant tried to rip out three times. Implant sewn back in three times. Implant removed. No breast on my left side. Goop for five months. Chemo. Being bald. Arimidex making me feel like bugs were biting me. Allergy to opiates making me itch. Heart almost stopping while having my port flushed. Whew! I was starting to feel worn out. I once again felt like I was a horse about to collapse at the finish line. Then the itching stopped. Glory Halleluiah ! It was a new year and I was not itching.

The other thing that was hard for me to handle, besides the itching, was that the new silicone implant was quite a bit higher than my other breast. I called Dr. Naman's office and talked to his assistant, Shana. "Don't worry. It'll take months for it to settle down in its permanent position. Everyday you need to lie on your stomach on your bed and push the implant down, about fifteen minutes if you can stand it. Also, you can push it down with your hand several times a day," she said.

"I'm afraid it'll start to leak or break or something..." I replied.

"No. You aren't going to hurt it at all. Just keep pushing it down. It's normal for it to look really high at first. You can push it inward too," she said.

Girlfriend advice: Here is a tip to put your mind at ease: Your implant , or implants, will be high and hard at first. Don't freak out! This is normal! Massage it. Push it gently down and to help make a nice cleavage push it inward. I got so upset when I saw that my implants were not at the same level right after surgery. After a few months they settled down and are now perfectly level. They are also exactly the same size. Yippeeeee!!!Thank you Dr. Naman!!!

I went back to see Dr. Pippas, my oncologist and I told him that I had once again experienced the horrible itching after surgery. He gave me the name of an allergist. He then asked me if I had recovered from the port flush that had knocked me out. I told him the truth. I said, "All I saw was bright light. But I could think. When I woke up my first thought was 'why did they wake me up?' I think I swallowed some of the light. I was euphoric for two days and then it just went away...." He just looked at me. He didn't say anything. I hoped that he believed me and I wondered if anybody else had ever told him that they had had a similar experience.

It was a new year. I went to the allergist and told him about all the misery I had experienced from itching after surgery. I was afraid that he was going to do a million tests and charge me a million dollars. He said, "There is no test to determine whether you are allergic to opiates. But, from what you have told me, I'd say that you are definitely allergic to opiates." He gave me a list of other drugs for pain that do not have opium in them. So my friend, the reason I have put so much in this story about itching is to save you some misery if you find that you wake up itching after your surgery. It just might be an allergic reaction to your painkillers that are opium based. Try painkillers that are not derived from opium and save yourself some major suffering.

In January of 2012, my oncologist told me that I was ready to have my chemo port removed. This is the same thing as saying, "I think you are cured." I was so happy to get the go ahead to have the port out. So I was off to see my surgeon Dr. Ken Smith, who had taken off my breasts. I had not seen Dr. Smith in about a year and a half. When he came in the door, he was grinning from ear to ear. I jumped up and hugged his neck. It was great to see him and I was so happy that he was happy to hear that my port could be removed. "When I take your port out I can give it to you so you can take a picture of it to put in your book," he said. I was so thrilled that he remembered I was writing a book about my cancer experience. So we set up my port removal surgery, which was surgery number fourteen.

I went back to the breast center and had the surgery on January 12, 2012. I was put into a semi-sleep. I asked Dr. Smith not to put any opium based painkiller in my IV. When I woke up I was not itching. Yippeeee!!! Walker drove me back to Fairy Ring Cottage and in a few hours I felt completely normal. I took two Tylenol just in case I started hurting, but I never hurt one bit. Good ole Dr. Smith!

For Valentine's, Walker took me on a one night trip to St. Augustine, Florida. We were trying so hard to get back to a normal marriage, a marriage that included sex and excluded cancer. We made a little progress. We had a really good time just hanging out together. We ate lunch at the Casa Monica Hotel. We walked around the historic district eating ice cream cones. We went to lots of little shops and Walker didn't even complain. We went into the old cathedral where my Pacetti ancestors had prayed for hundreds of years. We knelt and prayed. I prayed for a return to normalcy.

I continued to pray, "Holy Spirit dwell in me," about twenty times a day. I figured that when I opened myself up for the Holy Spirit to dwell in me, that I was opening myself up to all sorts of good things. I wanted to be healthy in body, mind and spirit. There is a billboard in Columbus, advertising the John B. Amos Cancer Center. It says they deal with your "mind, body and spirit" That billboard was telling the truth. The John B. Amos Cancer Center healed me on all levels, which is hard to find in a medical facility.

I wanted to be peaceful, free from anxiety, slow to anger and slow to be hurt by people. I wanted to have lots of energy. I wanted to be free from all fear, especially fear of a recurrence of cancer and death. I wanted this book to be published so that I could help other women get through breast cancer. I wanted to lose weight and firm up. I wanted to have sex without pain. I just wanted to feel like a new and improved Suzan. The Holy Spirit knew my needs without me even listing them. He knows yours too. Simply pray, "Holy Spirit dwell in me," and be surprised when you wake up one morning feeling happy. Really truly happy!

THE ROAD BACK TO A NEW NORMAL.

Dear Girlfriend,

The road back to normalcy after having battled cancer is not an easy road. After I had my port removed in January of 2012, there were other issues to deal with. As you recall, I had been taking an estrogen inhibitor called Arimidex. When I got hot, Arimidex made me feel like bugs were biting me. My oncologist, Dr. Pippas, switched me over to Letrosole, I had bug bites at first, but after several months they went away. Needing to switch meds can be so discouraging, but don't give up. If you need an estrogen inhibitor keep experimenting until you find one that gives you no bad side effects. If your breast cancer is estrogen driven you need to take an estrogen inhibitor if your doctor thinks that will lower your chance of a recurrence.

Also, after doing a bone density test, it was discovered that I had osteopenia, which means that I have lost some bone mass, but I don't have osteoporosis yet.

Girlfriend advice: Just remember this. Taking an estrogen inhibitor and having your ovaries removed can cause you to lose bone mass. If you take a drug like Tamoxifen, Arimidex or Letrosole, make sure you have a bone density scan. This is called a Dexa Scan. This scan will let you know if you need to take a drug such as Fosamax or Boniva to stop your bone loss. If you have bad side effects such as joint pain or swelling consult your doctor. At the very least, if you are on an estrogen inhibitor, you need to do load- bearing exercise, such as walking, everyday. I walk up and down our main staircase twenty times a day! You also need to take calcium citrate with Vitamin D to strengthen your bones.

So, here I sit in my cozy kitchen where I started writing to you. I was diagnosed with breast cancer on December 8, 2008. Today is my birthday, November1, 2012. Today I am fifty-six years old. My journey through cancer surgery, treatment and reconstruction has gone on so far for three years and eleven months. But, I am still alive and still writing to you. My silicone implant that I have had less than a year has settled down and looks lovely. It feels very natural.

I have completely changed the way I eat to reduce my chances of another recurrence of cancer. I bought a cool little smoothie maker that just makes one individual smoothie at a time. Every morning I make a smoothie out of one percent organic milk (that's milk without hormones), blueberries, a banana and four tablespoons of ground golden flaxseed. Flaxseed is thought to inhibit inflammation. It has omega-3 fats that are thought to help prevent breast cancer. Flaxseed has lignans that may occupy estrogen receptors on cells to help reduce the chance of breast cancer. Eating smoothies for breakfast is fun and tasty.

I also have started eating as many green leafy vegetables as possible. The lowly Brussels sprout is a good cancer fighting food. If you spray some olive oil in a glass dish, pour in frozen Brussels sprouts sprinkled with low fat shredded Parmesan cheese and microwave for about five minutes, you have an excellent cancer fighting dish that is so easy, you can eat it everyday. Another important supplement that might help to prevent cancer is garlic. I cook with as much garlic as possible and I take garlic gel caps daily.

Besides eating flaxseed and lots of fruits and veggies and organic milk, I take a multiple vitamin, calcium citrate with Vitamin D and fish oil. Fish oil is thought to help prevent cancer with its healthy omega-3 fats. I have tried to cut back on white sugar and other white carbs. For instance, I eat sweet potatoes instead of white potatoes. I try to avoid fatty foods as much as possible. Fat cells may produce estrogen and estrogen is what I need to avoid.

I exercise daily. Getting my body back in shape is proving to be a real challenge. I have gained fifteen pounds over my cancer journey due to lack of exercise. Since I've had fourteen surgeries in three years I haven't been able to exercise like I wanted. You might end up in the same boat. There might come a day when you have healed from all your surgeries and you look in the mirror and say, "Who are you?" That's what happened to me. My body was as soft as jell-o and I had gained so much weight. But, girlfriend, you can't give up. I don't like going to a gym so I just exercise at home. I feel like mush all over, but getting back in shape can't be as hard as all those operations.

Next, I have stopped drinking alcohol. It is thought that more than one drink of alcohol a day can significantly increase your chances of having breast cancer. Since I have stopped drinking alcohol I drink grape juice in a wine glass or non-alcoholic beer. Grape juice is loaded with cancer fighting vitamins and non-alcoholic beer is just as tasty as beer with alcohol. Of course you don't get a buzz, but it can be very entertaining watching other people drink!

Another issue I had to face during these last steps of reconstruction and return to normalcy stage is my nipples. Holy Moly! What a strange thing to say to somebody! I don't think I gave one minute's thought to my nipples until I realized that they would be removed along with my internal breast tissue. Since I had so many things go wrong, it had been over two years since my bilateral mastectomy. That meant over two years with no nipples. I didn't think I would miss them until they were gone! Without nipples my breasts looked like a Barbie doll. I went to Dr. Naman to discuss their reconstruction.

You see, normally the center part of your nipple, the part that stands up, is created surgically. The best way I can describe it is to think of a small circle in the middle of your breast. Now imagine if that little circle had some cuts in it, like cutting a pie. Now imagine twisting the "pie" to make a little sticky uppy nippy part that is tacked up surgically. Voila! Now you see why I am not a surgeon.

But, I had had so much trouble with not healing, that Dr. Naman said, "Look, your skin is so thin. Maybe instead of doing more surgery to create the center part of your nipples (the part that stands up) we could find a real tattoo artist that could make a tattooed nipple that looks three dimensional." Somehow I just couldn't picture myself going into our local "Ink Wizard Tattoo" and explaining to some guy with sleeves down both arms that I needed to see his color chart for my nipples. Did I want

"Passionate Pink" or "Reckless Red?" Decisions.... Decisions.... What to do in such a situation.... I called my girlfriend, Suzanne. "No! You don't go to a regular tattoo parlor! You go to a permanent makeup place. Go to Wendy Irvin at "Permanent Cosmetics by Wendy" in Columbus." So that is what I did.

When I walked into "Wendy's" I felt like I was going into a very nicely decorated doctor's office. Wendy showed me photographs of nipples she had tattooed. I kid you not . They looked real. I took off my shirt and bra and lay down on the cushioned lounge type chair. "Now, first I'm going to put some numbing cream on the nipple area, to help with discomfort." I really was a little nervous. "Are you sure this isn't going to hurt? I thought getting a tattoo hurts." Wendy said, "Some people that have body art don't want anything for pain. They want to feel that they "earned" the tattoo. But I'll make sure you are as comfortable as possible." All I could think of was after everything I had been through, I had definitely "earned" this tattoo.

So after about thirty minutes she put on a mask and rubber gloves and picked up an instrument that resembled a dentist's drill. I had flashbacks to the day I first received radiation. I still had time to jump and run, but as always, Walker was there with me, so I just scrunched up my toes, closed my eyes and squeezed the arms of the recliner. I heard her instrument but I didn't feel any pain. Whew!

When it was all over Wendy let me look in the mirror, "Wow! They look real!" I was so excited. "You need to wash them gently with Cetaphil, apply this moisturizing cream and come back in six weeks for a final touch up," she said. I couldn't believe how real they looked. Now, of course they won't ever stand up when I get cold, but there are advantages to that. If I want to wear a thin shirt with no bra then I don't have to worry about my nipples showing through my shirt. I went home and just stared at myself in the mirror. Wow. My new breasts looked great, except for one thing. Scars. Dr. Naman had done a fabulous job of reconstructing both of my breasts, but the one that had endured staph still had some scars, because I had not kept the incisions moist after surgery with Vaseline or Aquaphor. My bad.

Girlfriend, if your skin is not having healing issues make sure you keep those incisions moist to prevent scarring!

I got online and started looking up everything I could find about removing mastectomy scars. Silicone creams and silicone strips were all over the web. I ordered both the strips and the creams, but they didn't help the scars one little bit. I saw online that some women have laser treatments to remove scars, but I watched a video of laser treatments online and that looked pretty invasive. Then I saw "needling" is being used very successfully to remove scars and wrinkles. I called Wendy up and told her what I had seen online. "Yes. What I do is just run the instrument over your scars with no ink. That stimulates your skin to produce collagen and makes the scars look better." I was so excited! "Can you needle my scars?" I asked. "We can give it a try!"

I went to Dr. Naman and told him I wanted to try needling and he had no objections. He was also very impressed with my nipple tattoos. "They do look very natural," he said. So when I went back for my six week touch up for my nipples, Wendy needled my scars. I have had them needled two more times since then and I am seeing improvement. I feel certain that they are going to look significantly better. And Girlfriend, if you want to get rid of those crow's feet you may have good luck needling them away!

So, here I am in the trying to get back to normal stage. My friend Molly said, "I think it's going to be a new normal." I think she was right. Having cancer has been tough. It has put my mind and my body through the wringer. My mind will never ever be the same. But that could be a good thing. I have come to realize that this stage of life on earth is very short. For that reason, I try very hard to do only what I really want to do with people that I really want to spend time with. I see each day as an opportunity to do something that I really want to do, like sitting here writing to you. I want to write to you. I want to help you survive breast cancer with as little suffering as possible.

My mind is completely different because I have been forced to really think about what it means to be a human being. Here we are out in the middle of for real nowhere on a rock that is traveling around a big ball of fire. Well, what the heck are we doing out here, billions of miles from nothing, in infinite space? I have no idea, except that we are meant to be here. God brought us into existence. If we were not meant to be here then we would not be here. But, what are we supposed to be doing here in the little bit of time we have been given? I don't have a clue unless it is to love God and love our neighbors.

I have come to the realization that it doesn't do one bit of good to pretend that I own anything here on this earth. When I die I can't take anything of this earth with me, not even my body, so how can I say I "own" anything. All I can do, at best, is to borrow or temporarily use the good things on this earth. I can't take anything at all with me when I go into the next stage of my existence. Borrowed at best... Borrowed at best... When I think that I can't keep anything of this earth, it helps to release me from wanting so many possessions. Maybe my time here will be better spent making good memories with loved ones than storing up things that can't go with me after I leave this earth.

My body will never be the same. I mourned for my breasts. I mourned for their beauty. I mourned for my body that had no scars. I mourned my flexibility after I became stiff from chemotherapy and a lack of estrogen. I mourned all that I was physically before cancer. How can I get past the mourning of what my body was before cancer? All I know to do is to continue praying that the Holy Spirit will dwell in me and give me direction. I pray that I will be directed towards a new and better life as I embark on life beyond cancer. Hopefully this life will include a new way of taking care of my body and mind and new work as a published author and speaker for women who are also trying so hard to survive cancer. Maybe one day we will meet in person. So like I said in the beginning, you won't be cured until your body is free of cancer, your mind has no fear and your spirit knows that life is truly eternal. Cancer cannot destroy the power of eternal life. It cannot destroy the power of the resurrection of Jesus Christ. I know now that I can live forever and cancer can't change that.

The day came when I went for my last appointment with Dr. Naman. I was being released . Wow! I should have been so happy that my ordeal was finally over, but I wasn't happy. I was sad. I was sad to realize that I would not be seeing Dr. Naman and all of his staff anymore. Debbie hugged me and I said, "I'll just have to come back for some more procedures just so I can visit with y'all. I really could use a good face lift!" We both laughed.

Cheryl said, "Mrs. Rivers I'm going to miss you. This is bitter-sweet." It was just that. Bitter-sweet.

I told Dr. Naman that I felt like I had been held in a fire for nearly four years. "You know it says in the Bible that 'He will come to judge like one who refines and purifies silver....' Do you know how a silversmith determines that a piece of silver is ready to come out of the fire?" I asked him. Dr. Naman said, "How? How does he know when the piece is ready to come out of the fire?"

"The silversmith knows that the silver is ready to be removed from the fire when he can see his reflection in the silver. I guess God is going to hold me in the fire until He can see Himself reflected in me."

But, I can see God reflected in the eyes of so many people that have been there for me on this handheld walk through breast cancer. My doctors and their staffs. My family. My friends. Strangers whose names I never knew. My girlfriends. My daughters. My husband. Walker held my hand through the whole walk. I can see God reflected in his eyes. You know what? I really do love that man....

POST SCRIPT, DECEMBER 2012

You know I am amazed at the resilience of the human spirit. I have witnessed so much human suffering in my life. But Christmas time is rolling around again. All over town people are decorating with beautiful trees that hold a lifetime of memories in their precious ornaments. Everywhere I go I hear Christmas music and I can feel excitement and anticipation of the celebration of the birth of Christ. If I could get on a space ship and go to the moon, I could look back at our little planet all alone in the vastness of infinite space, just nothingness far past what the human mind can comprehend. But do we panic at the thought of this, our reality? No. We live in hope. We hang our mistletoe wreaths. We mail our cards full of love and well wishes. We keep the faith that we are out here on our little rock spinning around our big ball of fire because God wants us to be here and He will take care of us.

I make out my shopping list. I look up the ingredients for Waldorf salad. Again. I shop for the best apples I can find. Again. The earth just turns around. Again. And again. And again....I have faith that God has put me here and He will take care of me....

Finis

ABOUT THE AUTHOR

Suzan Rivers has worked for many years as a librarian, reading teacher, dramatic storyteller and puppeteer. Suzan is also a much sought after and very humorous speaker. She hopes that her story will make surviving breast cancer easier for other women.

She lives in Macon, Georgia with her husband Walker, a consulting forester. She has three daughters in college.

TO CONTACT SUZAN RIVERS:

www.facebook.com/suzan.rivers.1

www.amazon.com/author/suzanrivers

www.smashwords.com/profile/view/suzanrivers

WHAT OTHERS ARE SAYING ABOUT *"DEAR GIRLFRIEND"- A HANDHELD WALK THROUGH BREAST CANCER*

"In this well written book, Suzan shares her journey through the diagnosis and treatment of breast cancer. She speaks to the readers just like she would to her best girlfriends-- from the heart. This is a must read for all breast cancer patients . I will definitely recommend this to all mine."

Teresa Luhrs, M.D.

"Suzan Rivers provides something for everyone with her new book about surviving Breast Cancer. Her candid account of the journey she and her family took through this disease offers comfort to fellow survivors and those who love and care for them. Suzan also shines a critical light on the healthcare system, providing us with insight about what it's really like on the other side of the white coat. Amazingly, the author handles such a heavy subject with a light and humorous narrative that will truly make you laugh out loud. Cheers to Suzan Rivers for surviving cancer with grace and sharing her story with generosity."

Vincent Naman, M.D.

"Suzan Rivers' story underlines the cardinal rule for every cancer patient: each journey through cancer is unique. A successful cancer survivor refuses pat answers, questions continually, and leaves no stone unturned. Her "Dear Girlfriend"- A Handheld Walk Through Breast Cancer *will serve as a valuable guidepost for many women who face the challenge of breast cancer."*

Andrew W. Pippas, M.D.

"As a nurse, I strive to provide my patients with the information and resources they need to navigate from Breast Cancer diagnosis through survivorship. One area that I am unable to provide insight is that "first hand" experience…what does surgery, chemo, and radiation feel like? What happens to your heart and spirit each step of the way as you go through the process? I thought Suzan's book provided this so eloquently, so thoughtfully, and so respectfully. She tells us that while tears may be a normal part of the process, so

is laughter. Suzan offers that peer-to-peer support that only people sharing a similar experience can understand. I believe survivors who are prepared from every angle to fight Breast Cancer will have better outcomes physically and spiritually, and I think this book will open doors for women to seek that support that is so very much needed."

Lori Moser, RN, MSN, OCN, CBCN

"A no-holds barred look at a real live breast cancer survivor's journey through treatment and her tips for survival for those who come later to join this sorority. It's like "Steel Magnolias" for breast cancer."

Kenneth Smith, M.D.

"Suzan Rivers pulls back the curtain on breast cancer and sheds light into every dark corner of the disease. By unveiling the mysteries of the diagnosis and treatment process she helps other patients dispel their fear of the unknown. Suzan recounts her ordeal with humor and humility and keeps you laughing all the way. Congratulations to Suzan for conquering her Goliath and for using her talent to provide this wonderful gift to other breast cancer patients, survivors and their loved ones."

E. Mac Molnar, Jr., M.D.

17469014R00111

Made in the USA
Charleston, SC
12 February 2013